I'm so glad that God led Bill to put his updates from Crystal's bout with breast cancer into this wonderful book. Bill is a good husband, father, grandfather, coach and son-in-law. The View From the Front represents his experience from all these perspectives. You will be blessed by this family's heavy hearted daily walk during those tough months. As Crystal's father, I've been able to walk in peace over these years because of God's promise given to me on the day of her surgery. I pray this book will open doors for Bill to personally share this wonderful story with others who may need encouragement.

Billy J. Crosby, Pastor Emeritus, Summer Grove Baptist Church, Shreveport, Louisiana

A View From the Front gives us all an inside look at what it is like to face difficulty with a Big God in view. Bill's words will remind you that God is in your past, present and future. You will find yourself moving back and forth from tears to cheers. As you read through the pages of this book, you will discover that recovery, healing and spiritual growth all can come together during trials in life.

Jeff James, Pastor, Green Valley Baptist Church, Hoover, Alabama

Bill and Crystal have been the model of Christian faith and endurance throughout this ordeal. The View From the Front chronicles their journey and will provide hope to others who are having to walk the same road. I am grateful for their courage in sharing their story so that others may draw strength. Bill and Crystal are the embodiment of 2 Corinthians 1:3-4, "Blessed be the God and Father of our Lord Jesus Christ, the Father of mercies and God of all comfort, who comforts us in all our affliction, so that we may be able to comfort those who are in any affliction, with the comfort with which we ourselves are comforted by God."

Philip Gunn, Speaker of the House, State of Mississippi

The View From the Front is a wonderful testimony to the faithfulness of our extraordinary God in the lives of Bill and Crystal. As you read their story, you get a front-row seat to the grace of God being lived out before your very eyes. Bill and Crystal's life long confession of faith in Christ is put through the fire and comes out shining with the rare beauty of those who truly know their God and have found Him to be more than faithful.

Lisa Gunn, wife, mother of four

At a time when Bill and Crystal needed encouragement, they were the ones providing the encouragement to others. Bill's updates, compiled here in The View From the Front, would have me crying one moment and ready to hit the field the next. I am so thankful they allowed us to be a part of this big game with them.

Patrick Nix, Head Football Coach, Scottsboro High School, Scottsboro, Alabama

It's more than friendship. The profound impact the Gray's have made on our family began before Crystal's diagnosis. So, I wasn't surprised when her cancer journey became another example of how to live by faith. Although I talked to Crystal almost daily during that time, I would rush to read Bill's journal entries. It was the calm in the storm. His words were not just for them, they were for all of us. The View From the Front now gives you this opportunity. After reading this book, you will never be the same...

Krista Nix, wife, mother of four

The View
From the Front

A Family Faces the Reality of Cancer...
and the Promises of a BIG GOD.

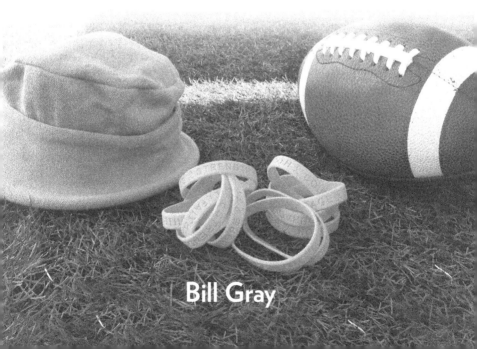

Bill Gray

Printed in the United States of America
Printed by Ebsco Media, Birmingham, AL
ISBN 978-1-937908-29-4
Printing Number 10 9 8 7 6 5 4 3 2 1

Cover Photo by Payton Gray
Editorial Work by Justin Burkhead
Design by: Rocky Heights Print and Binding, LLC.
This book is typeset in Adobe Caslon Pro

Additional copies of this book are available for sale online at
www.theviewfromthefront.com
Website Sponsored by Chronicle Studio

Amazon.com
....

To contact the author send correspondence to:
theviewfromthefront@gmail.com

Dedicated to Crystal

After watching you face this battle head on...
whether in the blue hat, or the hot wig,
or with the salt n pepper hair...
you have taught our entire family how to
stay strong in the eye of the storm.
You have been an inspiration, not only to me...
but to so many who have followed your journey.

As the scripture reminds us in Proverbs 31: 28 - 29,

Her children arise and call her blessed;
her husband also, and he praises her:
"Many women do noble things,
but you surpass them all."

It has been my privilege to have
The View From the Front.

Love you...

Table of Contents

Preface

For a wife, and family, that has always been private...we sure went public in a hurry. When Crystal was diagnosed with Cancer, we had a lot of family and friends that cared and wanted to know details. Details...so they could pray. Details...so they could help. Details... so they could be a part of our journey.

A teammate. A Team. Team Crystal.

So, what started out as journal entries on the CaringBridge website to keep our family and friends in the loop, quickly became an outlet for me to cope with the reality of my wife having breast cancer...and all the treatments that were to come. Whether it was early in the mornings, or late at night, I found comfort and strength in front of the computer relaying an update...and bragging on my God. Eight months after hearing the words "You've got Cancer", the updates were finished. The result is this book...or collection of God's Promises, that we placed our faith in as individuals and as Team Crystal.

During the time of this writing, our family of five had a calendar full of activities and commitments, much like I am sure your calendar looks today. My career path had taken me to work for a community bank, based in Tuscaloosa, Alabama but with my responsibilities keeping me in the Hoover area. Crystal was doing her thing as a stay-at-home mom and engulfing herself into everything our children were involved in both at school and church. Let me give you an idea of what our five children had going on during this season of our life.

Brittany, our oldest child, was a nurse at St. Vincent's Hospital in Birmingham, and newly married to Justin, who was in Beeson Divinity School while serving as a pastor of a small, local church. Briana, our second child, was finishing up her Family Studies degree at Samford University and just happened to be living at home during this time. Austin, our third child, was beginning his senior year at Bessemer Academy. He had just transferred to BA during that summer from Spain Park High School in Hoover. Payton, number four in line, was beginning his sophomore year at Spain Park. Both Austin and Payton were playing football that fall. Finally, Bailey, our youngest child, was entering the eighth grade at Berry Middle School, and a cheerleader. Get the idea of what our calendar looked like?

Although I was no longer coaching football when Crystal went through this journey, it didn't mean I wasn't ready to relate this battle to the many experiences we have had as a family in and around the football field. Crystal will be the first to tell you...and then my five children next...that they have a football coach for a husband...and father. That is all I will ever be in their eyes, and for good reason.

Crystal has never been happier in her life than when she was a mother to over one hundred college players. So, to make this collection of thoughts an encouragement to her first and foremost, it seemed natural to sit in front of the computer and go back to that time when we all smiled...regardless of the score.

As you read this book (and I use that term lightly), my prayer is that it will be an encouragement for the person whose hands are turning the pages. You may or may not be going through Cancer, that doesn't matter. You may or may not have a loved one experiencing their life being turned upside down. One thing is common for all of us...Life is tough. Life is hard. Life is a journey with so many Ups... and unexpected Downs. It would be my privilege to "coach you up" and brag on My God as you read.

One

You've Got Cancer...

Sunday, July 12

Everyone,

If you are getting this update, then you fall into one of the following categories: a family member, a close friend, a fellow church member, an old friend who we have recently heard from, an encourager we have heard from in the past few weeks, a co-worker, a neighbor, an extended family member, a prayer warrior, someone we have the utmost respect for or just someone who allowed us to have your e-mail address! Either way, you can figure out which category, or categories you fall into. I have tried not to leave anyone out who asked to be kept up to date. However, if you talk with someone and they want to be on this list, please let me know. Also, if you want to be excluded, then I can understand that as well. Suffice it to say, all of you are important to the Gray family. Please know up front that we know EVERYONE of us has struggles to face in this life. Some of you can relate to what Crystal is going through because of your own battle. Some of you have experienced far worse in your family. Some of you have shown us more compassion than we showed you. Some of you have encouraged us with your steadfastness and strength. We are very blessed to have felt your prayers and thoughts during the past few long weeks. Phone calls and cards have come out of the 'wazzu!' Thanks much.

Here is where we are as we begin the big week. Crystal goes to see the hematologist/oncologist on Tuesday (July 14th) afternoon to get the results of her barrel of blood work (I have never seen so many containers of blood in two hands). If they think her blood is where it needs to be (she was determined to be anemic last week) then we 'think' her surgery will be this Thursday (July 16th).

All the scans, x-rays, MRIs, tests and such have come back to show that it appears her cancer is localized to the left breast (first time I've ever typed that). We are praying that during surgery the surgeon will not find any cancer in her lymph nodes. As many of you know, she has Ductile cancer, which is the best of the breast cancer types.

Our surgeon is Dr. Philip Fischer. He did my hernia surgery in January, which may not give you much comfort (he recognized me when I dropped my drawers). He told us the bad news about as caring as anyone possibly could on that tough day. He talked of how God is Sovereign and how he doesn't understand why these things happen but he believes that it will 'work for good' because of God's promise in Romans.

Dr. Fischer, of course, was referencing **Romans 8:28** where we find, *"And we know that all things work together for good to them that love God, to them who are the called according to His purpose."* Not sure how the words "you've got cancer"...and *"work together for good"* can come together...but He does! So, we will 'tee it up and kick it off.' We will covet your prayers. We will hold fast to the promise a sweet doctor told us in a cold, sterile evaluation room.

"And we know..." Now that is good medicine!

Giving you... "my view from the front."

– Bill

Two

Floating Iron

Monday, July 13

Too many times, we turn to it last. Too many times, we don't unleash the power that it truly can have on us as believers just going through this thing called life. Too many times, we are sitting with the power, strength, and comfort... just turned off.

But not this time...so...

We ask that you pray for Crystal. Pray that she will be comforted by God's love and care. Pray that she will be able to feel a supernatural power while she is in the hospital. We know that He is the great physician.

Pray for Dr. Fischer and for her plastic surgeon. Pray for their steady hands, their sharp minds, for them to have divine direction, and for their intuition to know what they need to do once in the operating room. You can also pray that they get a good night's sleep on Wednesday evening.

Pray for the Gray kids. They have been so strong during this walk. They have all handled it differently and according to their personalities. Brittany has been the medical sounding board since she has the experience of being a St. Vincent's nurse. Briana has studied about some of the things Crystal is experiencing and has helped take the 'edge' off at home with the siblings. Austin has shown more compassion to his mom in the past month than in the past two years (he does have a sweet side). Payton wants to know why a doctor worth his salt can't give us answers NOW. Why the wait? Bailey is hanging in there. She has heard more from the phone conversations than most rising 8th graders. She understands everything that is going to happen. She is ok...until Crystal is not ok.

Pray for Crystal's recovery as well. She is going to have a double mastectomy and this will make it a tough surgery. She has fought long and hard trying to decide which route to go in this operation. She feels that this is the best thing for her, not only now but down the road also.

Things will be different for her after Thursday. She will be able to see her shoes for the first time since middle school. She will be able to wear more t-shirts. She will still be BEAUTIFUL to me. As some of you know, she is thinking about writing a book. I don't know if that will ever get off the ground but she does have her title set..."You Are Not Your N......." (I will let you fill in the last part). I am not sure how many churches will invite her to speak with that title but it will catch some attention in the bookstores.

Remember *2 Kings 6:6-7* and the story of the floating iron? *The man of God asked, "Where did it fall?" When he showed him the place, Elisha cut a stick and threw it there, and made the iron float. "Lift it out", he said. Then the man reached out his hand and took it.*

Floating iron? Really? He's God...why not?!

Finally, thank you again for all your prayers, cards, phone calls, thoughts, smiles, and hugs. We are trusting that the Lord will allow Crystal to be another success story in the battle against breast cancer. We are trusting that she will be able to help someone else get through this diagnosis. We are trusting that "our axe head" will float in the river this week, that God will provide for us a miracle – and if not, that we will still be faithful in trusting Him with this surgery and recovery.

I never thought I would see a pink bracelet on my wrist when telling the time. I never thought I would hold my wife's hand when the doctor said, "you have cancer." I never thought our life would suddenly become more chaotic than normal. I never thought I would see my wife receive so many signs of love and support.

Although there are so many things that have happened that I can say 'I never thought'...I do know NONE OF THIS surprised our Heavenly Father. HE IS IN CONTROL! HE IS FAITHFUL! IT'S GAME WEEK! TIME TO DO WHAT WE DO! THE GRAY'S LOVE YOU!

Thanks for letting me share what it looks like from... "my view from the front."

– Bill

Three

Pink Bracelets

Wednesday, July 15

I had something happen at work today and a coworker said, "be careful what you wish for." Well, after both Crystal and I were somewhat disappointed in having the surgery postponed last week... we were told today that "it is a go for Thursday." Her blood (iron level) looked better with the numbers rising. No other sign of anything to be concerned about. Crystal has found out quickly that the Bruno Cancer Center loves to look at your blood. Again, be careful what you wish for.

I am sure that at some point Wednesday night or Thursday morning we will be looking for someone to come around the corner and "postpone this thing!" I am going to give you the pertinent information first and then maybe give you some thoughts I have later. That way those of you that don't want to read the long version can still get the particulars. I have quickly found that this is one avenue for me to get some relief. So, thanks for bearing with my writing.

Crystal will be at St. Vincent's Hospital at 5:00 am this Thursday, July 16th. We expect her to be one of the first in line so that would put her in surgery around 7:00 or 7:30 am (now you know how they run you through like cattle if you have ever been in pre-op that early in the morning). The surgery we think will be about 3 to 4 hours, so she should have a very long morning. Thank you in advance for your prayers during the morning hours (I know a few on this list that might not even be up at that time of day!). I am hoping we can use Briana's computer to get some info out during the day on Thursday if we can find Wi-Fi... whatever that is. That is what we know at this point.

There are some other things we know at this point. One is that we have some Division I friends!! We have an All-American Family!! Our family is amazed at how caring and concerned and practical everyone has been...and we haven't even gotten to the hospital yet. Another thing we know is that I have had so many people say how God will put people in your path that you need at just the right time.

Let me tell you an example of that. We were taken out to eat by a sweet couple that we have gotten close to this past year and the wife gave Crystal a piece of paper with a name and number on it of a lady who had the exact same procedure done not too long ago. Not only that, but the lady's doctor was our doctor, Philip Fischer. (Remember, he is OUR doctor. Don't forget I had a procedure done as well not long ago. However, I didn't get this kind of response.) Please remember that name...Fischer. Pray for him.

Anyway, back to the story because there is more. So this friend of ours met this lady while in the hospital with her husband. Her husband, our friend, was having a procedure done and the lady on the note was a nurse at the hospital. So not only does she have first hand knowledge of the surgery Crystal is facing (with the same doctor) but she sees it from the eyes of a nurse. Now that in itself would be cool but there is more. This particular nurse had inquired about the "pink bracelet" on our friend's wrist and who it was for. Of course, it was for Crystal!

If you know anything about us, we really don't think things 'just happen.' ***Psalms 147:5*** says, ***"Great is our Lord and mighty in power; His understanding has no limit."*** This didn't 'just happen.'

When our fellow bankers started wearing those pink bracelets for Crystal last week, God knew that this nurse was going to inquire and get her contact info to Crystal by way of our friend. Do you see how He works? Do you understand that He is control? Do you see that nothing is too small or too big for my God? Do you rely on that promise as you traverse through life? Does it give you comfort? Do you share that comfort with others?

Let me add one final piece to this story. Our friend, the husband, who was in the hospital for the procedure...he is the one who ordered the pink bracelets for our bankers!! Now THAT'S MY GOD!! Did you follow what I just typed? God ordained it by putting the desire to order pink bracelets for Crystal in our friend's heart! Some of you will understand when I say, "that is a bread-breaking moment even Gideon would smile at."

So as I close tonight, we are trusting God because He already knows the outcome of Thursday. We are trusting Him to provide Crystal with strength because He knows what she is going to face. We are trusting God with the doctor's wisdom because He knows what they will find. It is still very hard for Crystal and our family, but not as hard because we know He already knows!!

I apologize for being so long in verse...but that is "the view from the front."

   – Bill

Four

Game Day...

Thursday, July 16

Team Crystal, let me give you a quick update on Crystal. After arriving here at 6:00 am this morning, she has just gone into surgery at 1:00 pm. We aren't expecting to have any news for several hours. Thank you for your continued support and prayer. I must admit, it was pretty tough to see her being rolled away from me and into the surgery holding area. Crystal wanted me to relay that she can definitely feel God's "Warriors" lifting up prayers on her behalf. While you are lifting up Crystal, I would ask that you lift up Nancy and her family today. She is a lady we have never met, but we know she is loved. She is a lady who had surgery at St. Vincent's this morning and her family and friends are grieving as I type. Those of you that know Crystal's father won't be surprised that he has already had "church" in the waiting room with them. There is "power" (immediate power) in prayer.

Later that Day

Team Crystal, we are still sitting and waiting...sitting and praying...walking around and wondering...walking around and praying...visiting and praying...praying and waiting. I think you get the picture of what is happening today at St. Vincent's. Crystal went into surgery at 1:00 pm. We don't expect to have much more info until much later in the afternoon. We covet your prayers and your care and your friendship. A stormy morning has turned into a cloudy day in B'ham. However, we can't help but feel like "it's beginning to rain!" We are looking to the heavens!!

Even Later that Day

Team Crystal, it is now 4:45 pm and we have just heard from the surgeons. Crystal came through the surgery well. She did good. She played the game hard! Dr. Fischer said that she didn't need any additional blood, which we were concerned about last week. Her vitals looked good and her blood pressure was in good shape. There was one area he said disappointed him...she did have cancer in her lymph nodes on the left side only. He had to go back in and remove "quite a few" of them. This doesn't mean anymore than what it says. It will be a few days before they will know exactly how far along the cancer is and the reality of the stage. We are holding on to the statements the doctor made from day one..."even if it is in the lymph nodes, I still think you will be a stage one or two." This diagnosis will determine the type of treatment and the amount that is used (chemo or radiation or a combo of each) once we get her to that step.

Hold on...they are calling me to the phone...Ok, I am back. The nurse just said that she is recovering well. She won't be very coherent for the remainder of the day because she needs to be "out of it" because of all she has gone through. Otherwise, she would be in a lot of pain. It has been a long day for everyone but none more than Crystal. The sun will come up tomorrow although I have felt somewhat like Joshua today as it has seemed like "the sun was standing still" for most of the day today.

Joshua 10:13, "...So the sun stood still and the moon stopped..." We have been in a room all day with so many lifting up prayers. Wonder... just wonder...if God might have been listening again today? Just like He did to Joshua. Thanks again for ALL the prayers and petitions. In reality, probably only the first quarter has been played. There is still the recovery, the treatment, and the CURE!! I have always wanted players who played hard from start to finish! I have a wife who is playing this game hard during the opening quarter!! As a family, we will start the second quarter tonight and make sure we are still playing strong.

This really puts a lot of things in life into perspective. The game is still on. The game has already been decided...we are going to be "dancing in the showers" after this one is played. Thanks for being in the stands.

All day long...that has been "the view from the front."

– **Bill**

Five

I See it on Your Face

Friday, July 17

Well, we closed it down! We were one of the first in the waiting room yesterday morning, and we were the last to leave last night. A very long day before we got to see Crystal after getting to her room from recovery.

Ever woke up to see a number of people surrounding your bed... with a look of concern on their faces? "I just don't want it to have spread to my lymph nodes" was one of the last things Crystal said before surgery. Well, how do you hide the truth? You can't on your face!

As Crystal woke up, and love was showered upon her, the "truth" was still evident on my face – at least according to her (I would never be any good at playing cards). Even though she was still "a bit off " from the anesthesia, she knew. She could see the concern on my face. Or maybe it was in my eyes. Either way...she just knew.

How do you tell someone who just spent hours in surgery... that it is worse than expected? I haven't had much practice in that.

How do you tell someone how thankful you are that they made it through surgery...that they did so good...yet, that the battle they face is much more than anticipated? Again, not much experience for me in that area.

How do you look at your wife through tears in your eyes and 'coach her up,' all the while wishing that you could take her place?

The locker room after a hard fought battle...regardless of the scoreboard...is eventually the same. When the noise has died down... the tears have been wiped...and the showers turned off...it is always the same. The faces tell the story. Those that gave it all they had on the field are exhausted. Those that paid the price every snap...are worn out. Those that displayed determination and strength just have that "look." You can see it on their face.

I Chronicles 16:11 tells us where to "look." It says, *"Look to The Lord and His strength; seek His face always."* In the days ahead, those standing around that bed last night (and most importantly, the one under the sheets) will need to "look" to the Lord for strength. It looks like this one will be a tough battle.

Crystal knew that there was more to the surgery than hoped for... because she saw it on my face.

The battle will be won...and much more than we will hope for...as we look to the face of our Lord. We will see it in His face.

Let's face it...that's "my view from the front."

– **Bill**

Six

Beautiful Feet

Saturday, July 18

Let me start by saying, we put a man on the moon, we have chicken biscuits, we have microwave ovens, we have ethanol gas, we have arena football, we have (had) tear-a-way jerseys, we have lazy boy recliners. So why can't we get hospital furniture that you can sleep on?! I think that company should be recession proof!! But enough about me.

We have almost completed day three of this journey and I wanted to give you an update on Crystal. Thank the Lord that day three was better than day two. I am sure that there will be days where we step backwards, but as of now we have stepped in the right direction.

Crystal had a little fever this morning (and last night) so the doctor decided to keep her another day and monitor her. This evening her numbers are better so we are planning on "blowing this joint" tomorrow. Her pain has been tolerated thanks to her pain medicine. It sometimes seems like the four hour periods are eight hours apart. The key is to get the meds BEFORE you need it (my public service announcement – at no charge).

Crystal walked up and down the hallway twice today. She is not ready to back-peddle yet, but she had pretty good form in the forty. Her time wasn't good enough to record…I think it was the clean new white house shoes courtesy of one of our dear friends. Since she is moving around some, this has enabled her body to start the healing process.

The other "big hurdle" today was getting the surgical bra (not the "bro" that you may have seen on Seinfeld)! I never knew it would take a court order to get the surgical bra she was supposed to receive after surgery on Thursday. I will tell you, court order or not, if a husband goes to the nurses desk and is "stern" in his directive…things can get done quicker. I didn't know those things were coming from overseas daily!!! You would have thought it was made out of gold. This has given her some comfort as she moves from place to place. It was a life-saver.

We can't help but continue to be uplifted by the kindness being shown to Crystal and our family. We are blessed. There have also been a number of things done "behind the scenes" that will always be in our hearts. Do you know that in addition to all the prayers being lifted up for Crystal on Thursday, we had some sweet friends who were "prayer walking" around the hospital without our knowledge? That is putting feet to your faith, literally. The Bible talks about *"how beautiful are the feet of those who bring good news" (Romans 10:15)*. Our friends, the prayer-walkers, must have beautiful feet.

Team Crystal will have their first home game beginning tomorrow. The second quarter has started well and we will continue the recovery process until her forty time is under 4.5. We know it is still early in the process but we have so much to look forward to and have been encouraged by those who have run these same plays before. Some have come by the hospital to show Crystal that better days are ahead. We have faith that this will happen. Thanks for everything from prayer to pink icing!

That is the "view from the front."

– **Bill**

Seven

...To Be a 1

Sunday, July 19

"Are you ready to go home?" That is how Crystal's day began. And all the people said, "Amen!" Dr. Fischer came in this morning and gave Crystal the green light to "blow this joint." It was good to get her home to a more familiar surrounding. I will say that the ride down Hwy. 280, although done hundreds of times before, seemed a little different. Our family was changed as this ride was being made. Something like this will change you in a lot of ways.

Crystal received some good medicine when she got home. It didn't take long for our bedroom to get crowded with children. She needed to have a "comforter of kids" around her (once today I even saw all four of my girls in the bed at one time watching part of a Lassie movie!). That is the good medicine she needed.

Crystal is ok as long as I don't forget the pain medicine schedule (her next pill is at 1:00 am this morning). She has gotten to rest today which has been good. Her body has been through so much over the last four days. She has been a trooper. She has faced this head on and has not backed down. Dr. Fischer will not have the exact results of the tumor or the lymph nodes until later this week... some more anxious days are ahead. In my former world, I would say that the opponent is doing some things defensively that they haven't shown before. They are taking chances and are blitzing quite a bit. This will cause them to make some plays...but be patient. Because of them taking chances, WE TOO WILL BEGIN TO MAKE SOME PLAYS!!

Cancer, throw your best punch, because we are fixing to go on the offensive!! I learned a long time ago that the best defense can be a good offense. Team Crystal is fixing to go on the offensive. We are now playing at home where we are tough! We are in the second quarter of this thing and know this cancer: we will fight for the entire four quarters. Hope you brought your lunch! We continue to be amazed at how God has "placed" people in our path during Crystal's walk. We are blessed to have you as a concerned friend, prayer warrior, intercessor, teammate, and behind-the-scenes playa!! Thanks from all of us. It has been amazing how people have been "led" to do certain things...needed things...at just the right time. Our God is Sovereign. He is in control.

I have to say before I close how much our children have done in this difficult situation. Their mother is a good teacher. Brittany (with Justin's support) has been a better nurse than any we had during our stay. The girl knows how to care. She knows what to do before it needs to be done. She, in a strange way, has been the guiding force for Crystal during some painful moments.

Briana has been an extension of Crystal through this. She has kept the food organized, the kitchen cleaned, and the siblings on schedule. She has been our communication central. Much of this site has been her doing. She has been a rock.

Austin has continued to be willing to do "whatever" is needed. He has helped so much with the things around the house that need doing. He was in charge yesterday when our "sump pump" (newly repaired sump pump) went out again. He was the man! He is the man (he is even soft and considerate).

Payton – Mr. P – has done so much to keep all of our spirits up, including Crystal's (you should have seen his "Patch Adams" impersonation in the hospital last night. You know, the glove over the head like a chicken? Funny stuff). Nobody cares like he does. He has always had such a tender heart.

And I can't leave out Bailey, my little girl who is not little anymore. She gave her dad a hug last night before bed that could melt the frozen tundra (she even initiated it). She has learned so much, seen so much, heard so much, and felt so much in the last several weeks. She is no longer a little girl. I am so proud of them all.

So, I finally got to the computer tonight as Crystal is in a deep sleep upstairs. I told her what our neighbor reminded me of this afternoon. He said "Bill, there is only two numbers that matter in this thing (we were talking about her stage of cancer). Those numbers are 1 and 0 (they have faced cancer head on with their son). 1 you live and 0 you don't. You do whatever is necessary to be a 1! He didn't know it at the time but he had just grabbed me by the nap of the neck. He was encouraging me to not waiver in encouraging Crystal. Our attitude is so important during this trial.

Can I close with a couple of other numbers for you? They are **Psalms 107: 28 -29, "They cry out to the Lord in their trouble, and He brings them out of their distresses. He calms the storm, so that its waves are still."** Today was as beautiful a day in July as you will ever see in Hoover, Alabama – blue skies, mid seventies, and low humidity. However, the sound you may have heard coming from our home today was for God to *"**calm the storm!**"*

Roll up your sleeves, Cancer, you are in for a fight. Team Crystal is going to make adjustments in the second quarter. We are going to "air it out." We are on the offensive. Our QB is and will always be... undefeated!!

That is our "view from the front."

– **Bill**

Eight

Adjustment's in Life

Tuesday, July 21

When an offense comes off the field they gather and talk. They talk about what worked and what didn't work. They talk about what the defense is doing and how they can attack when they get the ball back. Any offense worth their salt can make adjustments during the game. They make adjustments because they have prepared for anything that they may see. They have prepared for whatever is "in front of them." They make adjustments and they don't panic because they have "faith" in the team.

The same is true in my new profession. You start a relationship with someone because you believe in the individual behind the deal. You believe in the business with the product or the service. You believe that the individual will adjust when and if he has to make adjustments. You believe they are prepared for what is in "front of them." You believe that there will be better days ahead if you make some necessary adjustments today.

Today the surgeon called and gave us some much anticipated

news. He said that they removed a total of 13 lymph nodes from under Crystal's left arm and a total of 4 were cancerous. This was a good percentage for us! We were hoping for 3 or less but we will make "adjustments" because of what is in front of us. The size of the tumor is a little larger than we were expecting. We will make adjustments again because of what is in front of us. We will find out in the coming days the exact stage of her cancer. That is still out there somewhere in front of us. But you know what, we are ready. We will adjust.

Some adjustments are already being made. Crystal is adjusting to the discomfort of her drains that hopefully will be coming out soon. Can anyone out there get these out?!! Crystal is adjusting to sleeping on her back in a slightly inclined position. This is something she has never done. But she is making adjustments because that is what is in front of her.

Crystal birthed and raised five children. She always had them on a feeding schedule at night. She breast fed and would say that I "slept through most all of it." Well, she must be starting to pay me back.

We are now on a "medicinal schedule" and I set multiple alarms for multiple times at night. Sometimes we both stumble around and find the right medicines to take in the middle of the night. We adjust – because we have this in front of us.

I write this journal from time to time to help you get a small glimpse into our season of life. To hopefully help you face whatever is in front of you. But I have found quickly that this website gives us a glimpse into the faith of our visitors and the Goodness of our God!! Crystal and our family have joined a much too large community of those that have experienced cancer. We can now say that we have been there. She has found comfort from those who have walked the same road she is walking. I have always said that "unless you have been in the locker room and the huddle, you really don't know what it is all about."

I was on the other end of the phone today with a friend whose sister has just been diagnosed with breast cancer. You know, I could actually relate to what she was going through. I have now been there. Crystal can now assist others in their walk because she is there. That is what this world is really all about – assisting others with "their walk." As I was driving over Red Mountain today and listening to a voice mail, I was reminded that Gideon couldn't understand God's plan for him. Remember, God found him under a tree and told him of the great things that would be accomplished. *"When the angel of The Lord appeared to Gideon, he said, The Lord is with you, mighty warrior" (Judges 6:12).*

Gideon had an idea of how to get it done, but God had another plan, a plan that didn't make much sense at the time. However, it was a plan that not only would work but would be so much more of a victory than Gideon could ever have imagined. It also was a plan where only God would get the glory! Adjustments were made because of what was in front of Gideon. Adjustments that could only come from a sovereign God.

As I close, I pray that you will allow God to make the necessary adjustments in your life. I pray that you will find comfort in knowing that we don't have anything in front of us that He has not already experienced. He wants us to lean on him so we won't be "stumbling around" in the dark. He wants us to know that what He did on His "tree" was for ALL of us. We don't take lightly the kindness that has been shown to Crystal and our family.

When you hear of prayers that are literally raised up all over the country on behalf of your wife...that is big stuff ! That will make a fake eye cry!! We have found quickly that in Hoover people know how to cook food, grow veggies, bake, pick restaurants and deliver on time. Crystal will be the first to say we don't deserve this (our boys might argue though, they sure are enjoying this part of the deal). Thank you all.

Finally, I want you to know that "the view from the front" has not changed!! She is still beautiful!!

– **Bill**

Nine

Seeing the World

Thursday, July 23

"Elvis has left the building!" I never saw Elvis in concert but I have heard that expression on many occasions. You know when everyone would keep cheering and asking for an encore. They just wanted to see his "hips" one more time. However, the announcer would come over the intercom and say, "Elvis has left the building!" Well, in our own little world, today Elvis (I mean Crystal) left the building!! I took Crystal to the plastic surgeon for the first of many follow up visits. She got out into the world today...you go girl!

Now I won't tell you how long and difficult it was to get her up, showered, dressed, and out the door...but she did it...and on time too. I don't know how many of you have ever been to a plastic surgeon's office, but as I referenced last time, I have been in the locker room. I have experienced it. It is indeed different. There was one thing we ALL had in common while there...the finished product!

Crystal got one step closer to that finished product today when they removed two of her three "utters," or drains. Now before you raise an eyebrow to me, that is what she has been calling them, her "utters." So, she was "two for three" today (utterly ridiculous!). Not a bad average. We hope the other drain comes out next Tuesday. Then, she won't have to put them in her pants pockets anymore! Yes, she was putting them in her pocket to hide them and to relieve some of the pressure of them hanging. Anybody got a quarter (we seem to be getting more detailed with each journal entry)? The doctor said everything was on schedule and to "think about the finished product, and not get caught up in the early stages." We will come back to that statement.

After the doctor visit, we then went and had a sandwich for lunch. Now how about that? One week out of a major surgery and life change, and we are breaking bread in a sandwich shop full of "tennis moms." I was proud of her. I am just glad none of them asked her for change!! You know what, the turkey was just as good as she remembered. The hustle and bustle of people at lunch was just as fast as before. The sun was shining, the phones were ringing, the sweets were being boxed. It reminded me that life will go on...just a little differently for some.

Yesterday was her first minor meltdown. She got upset over a minor incident (a child got left without a ride, no big deal....) and some emotions came out that have been building up. I told her if anyone has a right to "melt it down" it would be her. No big deal. I was glad, in a way, that she showed some of those emotions. We will try to work our schedules out a little better so that won't repeat itself. Again, no big deal. If you know my wife, she wants to have a finger on the when and where of each child at all times. It isn't overbearing but just "momma caring." She is going to have to adjust a little over the next few months...just not yesterday.

You know there is always someone who is in more of a situation than you. I remember the scene in Jaws where they are in the boat at sea and they are comparing scars. Remember how they went back and forth trying to "one up" the last one. Well earlier this week, a friend of ours gave a kidney to his sister! He sacrificed his organ for the good of a loved one. He went through a major surgery and did it voluntarily. He will be off the golf course for several months because "he wanted to." We know this journey of ours is very tough and very serious, but there are journeys out there all over the place. Each day we are so humbled by the support our TEAM has shown for Crystal.

My friend's sister will have a healthier "finished product." Crystal's body, we believe, will have a healthier "finished product." Too many times we get caught up in the here and now. We need to think about the "finished product." Because of God's grace and mercy, we too can have a better "finished product." He voluntarily did that for us!! Elvis may have left the building...but our Savior is coming back! What a day that will be!! Will you be able to say, like Paul to Timothy, *"I have fought the good fight, I have finished the race. I have kept the faith" (2 Timothy 4:7)?*

Finishing up with..."the view from the front."
– Bill

Ten

And That's the Way It Is

Saturday, July 25

Those words used to come off the lips of the late Walter Cronkite. He would often close his broadcasts with, "and that's the way it is." Well yesterday was somewhat of a watermark day for Crystal. It was also a day when we realized finally – that this is how it is!

We began the day with our second consecutive day of getting up and getting dressed to face the outside world (two less "utters" made it a little easier for everyone). Crystal had a morning appointment with Dr. Fischer, our general surgeon. We have found over the last month that he is very "guarded" in his words. He doesn't want to put the "nail in the wall" until he knows for sure that is where he wants it to go. We went in wanting to know a couple of things: "How are the incisions looking?" and "Can you tell us what is the stage of the cancer?".

The area of the surgery is looking good and is on schedule for recovery. The other question was not answered the way we had hoped. Dr. Fischer said that Crystal's cancer is a STAGE 3-A because of the size of the tumor and the amount of lymph nodes affected. Now I am learning so much about this awful enemy but there is still so much to learn. However, I do know that 3 is not as good as 2 but A is better than B!! Crystal said after we left the office that she "did good by not crying." Sometimes you have to be careful what you ask. AND THAT'S THE WAY IT IS!

The other watermark for the day was that she slept WITHOUT the aid of Lunesta or pain pills!! Your prayers are reaching the KING. She has graduated, for the time being, to Tylenol and such. This is a big step. Now don't get me wrong, she is not ready yet to swim laps in a pool, but she is getting better day-by-day. This also made our night a little more normal. We were back to one alarm setting.

So, yesterday was a better day all in all. Sure we are disappointed in the stage. However, does the stage determine our attitude? Does the stage determine how much she fights? Does the stage determine how important LIFE is? Does the stage control our approach to each day? Absolutely not!! I heard the expression years ago – "and then some." Well, the hill will be just a little steeper. The fight just a little tougher. Our team will still attack the cancer – "and then some."

In football, when you have them down, you step on their neck (figuratively speaking of course)! If "that's the way it is" then now we know how to approach the next phase. She's getting better. The second quarter is moving on. We want to recover and have some momentum going into half-time. The VICTORY will only be that much SWEETER!

Now to this morning...

Crystal woke up today and for the first time outwardly expressed how she "wished it wasn't true. I want it to be like it used to be!!"

Now guys, that was tough for me. We had our moment in the quiet of this Saturday morning. We just sat on the bed and well, you can imagine. We have extended the embrace of our hugs over the last several weeks. (PSA...Hugs are good!). We regrouped and we are moving forward facing our day (I know there will be more "moments" to come).

I was reminded this morning what Max Lucado says in his book Facing Your Giants. He references *John 20:19, 22* by saying that *"God brings BREAD for the SOULS (Peace be with you) and He brings a SWORD for the STRUGGLE (Receive the Holy Spirit)."* Our family has been comforted by the BREAD that has been provided by our Heavenly Father (the pound cakes haven't been bad either). Our family, with Crystal in the center, has sharpened our SWORD for this struggle. God gives both to the desperate! As hard as it is sometimes to say... "THAT'S THE WAY IT IS!"

Have a great Saturday. I hope it is a watermark day for you and your family.

Again, "the view from the front."

– Bill

Eleven

One is the Loneliest Number

Monday, July 27

Numbers, numbers – everywhere there are numbers! Have you ever noticed your day is filled with numbers? Let me give you some examples from our world (stay with me). Yesterday was a "3 or 4" for Crystal. I asked her that question tonight. On a scale of 1-10, she was not ranking it very high. Sunday morning...in pain, wondering should we go see the surgeon to ask about the swelling. Sunday afternoon...four sweet visitors, but after they left...tears. Still uncomfortable with the pain. Sunday evening...no pain pills tonight, no sleep aids, just life after surgery. And a few more tears. So you can see why the day wasn't ranked very high. Numbers!

Today, work called me to T'town for most of the day. We spent the better part of five hours talking numbers! That is what you do in the banking industry. Talking numbers, charting numbers, predicting numbers, and planning and preparing for more numbers.

Get the picture of what we discussed in T'town...numbers! Regardless of the numbers, I am blessed to have a family of bankers who care.

Talked to Crystal on the phone on my way home. She went to the surgeon to check out her swelling. Thanks to a sweet friend for taking her while I was away. That, in itself, was a watermark for Crystal. If you know her, she is not one to ask for help...from anyone. Again, you go girl!

Her plastic surgeon asked her if she wanted the last utter taken out. I don't think he used those words, but that is essentially what he said. Her surgery still looked good in his eyes.

She is still on pace. Good news.

"So, do you want me to remove your drain?" All the people didn't say AMEN. Crystal said, "I don't know!" WHAT??!! The doctor asked her if she had "become attached to her final drain." One IS the loneliest number! I wasn't there, but if he wants to take your last utter out, then by all means, "let Calhoun have it!" After a couple of seconds of pondering, she relented. Drain number three is history!! (She was just afraid of some swelling occurring under her arm where her lymph nodes were removed. He told her it was time to part with the drain.) One lonely formally attached drain...gone! Numbers.

While on the way home from T'town, I got to talk some numbers with my oldest son. We got to have some very important conversation involving cadence. You know, snap counts! Calling plays at the line of scrimmage. Again, numbers...824!...335! You get the picture. Something only a father and his son can relate to...numbers. So tonight I asked Crystal to rank her day. She said "6 or 7!" A much better day. More numbers, but better numbers. Twice as good as yesterday. Music to my ears (makes a glass eye cry!).

It seems like for the last several weeks we can't get away from the numbers. Cancer in 1 breast. 2 breasts removed. Stage 3a. 4 lymph nodes. 5 children (plus Justin) hurting for their mother. A long 6 months. Numbers, numbers, numbers. Here are a couple of more examples and I will close. We have had over 2200 hits to this site in support of Crystal. We have had over 100 guest book entries to encourage my wife and family!! Those are amazing numbers. But as amazing as those numbers...words are so much better!! Words that stop you in your tracks. Words that lift you up. Words that light that fire inside your belly. Words that dry tears. Words that cause tears of joy. Words that bring back memories. Words that remind you of how fortunate we are as a family. Words that speak volumes.

Some of those words are: long ago friends, roommates, hang in there, I'm a survivor, praying for you, just found out about your battle, a hug for you, just want to see your face, you mean so much to me, your mom led me to the Lord, do you need anything, how can I help, know we are praying for you, I think of you constantly, you don't know me but, so many are pulling for you, mom look what they brought you, just wanted to know how she is, more food, remember when you were young, family, just wanted to check in today...

Psalm 107:29 talks about how God *"stilled the storm to a whisper; the waves of the sea were hushed."* That is how the Gray's feel when we hear and read your words. God speaks through your messages and calms our storm. He speaks to us in a whisper. I could go on and on about what your words have meant to us during the first half of this journey. My words...our words...seem so inadequate for the love my wife and family have felt from Team Crystal. All I know to say are two words....Thank You!

Quietly looking at... "my view from the front."

– **Bill**

Twelve

Square Peg into a Round Hole

Thursday, July 30

Where to start? Too much running through the mind to comment on all of it, but a few thoughts will make their way to the keys. I can't help but think that two weeks ago tonight we circled around Crystal in the hospital room and couldn't find the words for the moment. She looked like she had just gone five rounds with Joe Frazier! Her face was swollen, her eyes had some "gunk" all over them, her nose had tubes, and her chest was wrapped like a cocoon...not a pretty site.

She looked up at us as we looked down at her. One of those rare moments when words were not adequate at the time. Just a circle of love...with a quiver of children wanting to change places. It was like putting a square peg into a round hole...it just didn't seem to fit. Just for the record, Friday morning she looked so much better!

School registration took place this week. For the first time, Crystal wasn't standing in line signing up the kids. I took one during lunch one day, Briana took another one morning and one took himself. Now I must admit, in all the years of our kids going to school, this was my "maiden voyage" on the "sea of registration." I discovered there aren't many dads in line. I discovered there are way too many forms and books to read. I discovered you can feel out of place in a hurry...again, trying to put a square peg into a round hole...it just didn't seem to fit. Just for the record, I think everyone is registered for their appropriate grade with only one lunch period each!

Today was expansion day! Not like the NFL where a city does all it can to get a team. It was more like going to the plastic surgeon and beginning "the process." This was indeed like putting a square peg into a round hole...it fits where?! I will let you find your local breast cancer patient to get some explanation on that last part. Uncharted waters indeed (things are starting to "shape up").

I have found over the last several weeks and especially over the last few days that this cancer thing can really make you feel like your little world from before just doesn't fit right today. There are a lot of times when you feel words are not adequate at the time. There are a lot of times when you can feel out of place in a hurry. There are moments when you stop and stare at uncharted waters and realize it is all a part of the process.

I think if I was honest with you, I would say there are times when you want to take that "square peg of life before" and force it into this "round hole of life today". You know as well as I do that you can't do that. You can't look back at what was and expect it to change what is.

It is like the summer when I drove a tractor for my uncle and planted soy beans. You started a row by finding a tree at the far end of the field and concentrating on that tree. As you drove across that dusty field with the planter, your row was going to be straight as long as you didn't let your eyes leave "the tree." But the moment you looked back at what you had done before...at what was behind you... you realized the tree had seemed to move. Not only could you not locate the tree but your row was no longer straight. Looking back... didn't do much for what was forward and in front!

The same is true not only for cancer patients (and families) but also for each one of us. When we fix our eyes on "THE TREE", it is amazing how He can straighten our world out! When we feel like life has given us a round hole with a square peg, it is amazing how He can allow things to fit just right...like he planned it all along...if we just give it over to Him.

In *2 Corinthians 4:18,* we read *"so we fix our eyes not on what is seen, but on what is unseen..."* There are no waters that are uncharted for Him. There is no situation we can be in where we should feel out of place. And when words seem so inadequate at the time...that is when He speaks to us in a "still, small voice."

We are probably mid-way through the second quarter (recovery process) and as someone special told me today, "We are here coach, just put us in!" I don't know what our scholarship limit is but we have plenty of players who can get the job done on Team Crystal. It is because of those players, and their abilities, that Crystal and our family are able to "round off our square peg days."

Still the "view from the front"...

– **Bill**

Thirteen

Lazy Saturdays... No Way!

Saturday, August 1

"What do you want to do today?" Seemed innocent enough when I asked that question this morning. You know, lazy Saturdays when you really don't have anywhere you have to be. Aren't you glad when those days come along?

At the Gray house, it usually means yard work! My boys don't always look forward to Saturday mornings. However, I was asking this question to Crystal. "Let's get you out of the house and get a change of scenery today." But she wasn't sure she wanted to do that, so the boys and I went outside and attacked the yard. Sorry boys but Grandpa trained me all too well. Saturday mornings mostly meant work, then play!

Before we started on the yard, I watched as two of my neighbors talked about something they had in common. They both have recently lost their jobs. So many during these last few months have fallen into this category. As we have found out with this cancer, it is always good to talk with someone who really knows what you are experiencing. On our street it seems like this job conversation has gotten too large of a group lately. What they have in common is trusting God with the future! Not much different from our cancer support group.

Doing the yard gave Crystal time to figure out what she wanted us to do this Saturday. Careful what you ask for. There is no "us" in watching me clean the kids' tub!! Brillo pad? How do you turn it on? I have seen her start nesting when she was about to be birthing a baby. But I didn't know breast cancer would make her want our house to be spotless! So, if you come to our house tomorrow you can now shower in a very clean tub. I was up to my elbow in some blue gunk. It is amazing what can make a wife happy.

We did finally get out of the house for a late lunch at her favorite restaurant...Superior Grill. Fajitas and chicken soup are good for the soul! And after lunch we went to Home Depot, which was to pay her back for the tub!! We would have gone looking for another post-surgery bra, but some place called "Touching You" was closed – thank the Lord! So, today was a big day for my wife...lunch and some fertilizer! You can see she is making progress. I will think twice before asking her next Saturday what she wants to do.

The date circled on our calendar now is next Tuesday, August 4th. On that afternoon we will meet with Crystal's oncologist. I am sure at that time we will get a "game plan" for the third quarter of this game. There really is not an hour that goes by that we are not thinking of that meeting. Whether cutting grass, scrubbing tubs, eating fajitas, welcoming friends, rising in the mornings or turning in at night...we are thinking about the game plan! You know...we know...and others have known...that God has already written the plan. He just wants us to step out in faith and exercise the plan.

I can't help but think of *Jeremiah 29:11*. That verse has been mine and Crystal's verse since we got married. It talks about how Jesus has a plan for our life. It is a plan to prosper us and not to harm us. It is a plan for a hope and a future. We have quoted that verse hundreds of time. We even have it on a beautiful serving platter from our "Muddlers S.S. Class." Yet it is still tough at times. You know what I mean? Some of you, like us, have been there from time to time in your life.

Sometimes on Saturday night, I will go to the man cave and get my fix of the Gaithers (some of you can't quite picture that). There is a song that has a line *"I believe. Help thou my unbelief. I walk into the unknown trusting all the while."* It is when someone quotes *Jeremiah 29:11* to me in a voice mail...or calls Crystal and talks about the cancer that they have whipped...or writes of a victory on this website...or surprises me in a bookstore and tells me an encouraging word (with a hug)...or just drops her a timely card. Those are players on Crystal's Team that *"help thou our unbelief!"*

Know that the sole purpose of this journal is to "help thou the unbelief" of someone who is going through a tough game like Team Crystal is playing this fall. Keep the faith! Play hard! Execute the plan!

That is tonight's "view from the front."

– Bill

Fourteen

Hearing vs. Listening

Tuesday, August 4

Have you ever had someone look you in the eye and speak to you in plain English…and you understand not? As hard as you tried, you just couldn't hear. There is a difference in "hearing" and "listening." Maybe I was hearing today…but I just couldn't listen! Some of it was the fact that I was hearing words that I have never heard before… words that just sound bad. Words that seem to just zap you of your energy. Crystal's oncologist was speaking from the heart. She was using plain English. There really just wasn't any way to "sugar coat" the Game Plan. It is what it is.

Crystal and I went to get the Game Plan today for the third quarter. We are closing in on half time. Shortly we will be going into that locker room to "make adjustments." The third quarter will be so much longer than the second! Get off your feet…rest…grab an orange…hydrate. "Listen" to the adjustments. It's very important to attack the first five minutes of the third quarter. We have prepared for a moment like this! As Crystal has reminded me, "We thought winning a football game was tough! That was NOTHING!!"

Here are the particulars. Things to look for in the third quarter. She will start her chemo treatments on August 25th. She will be introduced to "the Red Devil" (that is what they call the stuff). "Red Devil" meet "Prayer Warriors!" She will have one treatment every other Tuesday for four weeks. Then, she will progress to one treatment, every week, for twelve weeks. Then comes radiation, five days a week, lasting four to six weeks! Are you listening? See what I mean? I was hearing but I wasn't listening. What a third quarter?! This thing is going to stretch into February and March. Guys, get off your feet!

Just a few more items. She should be losing her hair after the second treatment. Something tells me we will have some "unique" birthday pictures in September. We left the hospital with "wig brochures." Never would have imagined that I would be sharing "wig brochures" with my wife. Also, she will be taking a multitude of pills, a stack of prescriptions. I think there are even pills for pills! She reminded me that she has gone from a healthy lady who "never took prescriptions" to having her own mini pharmacy. Finally, she wanted to schedule her treatments on Tuesdays. We have football games to see on Mondays and Fridays. Mom can't miss her boys play!! Again, you go girl!!

Over the last few days, I have been reminded repeatedly what it means to "listen." I have "listened" when scripture has been quoted and applied to our unique situation. I have "listened" when God has amazingly placed people (seemingly from out of nowhere, or right under our noses) in our paths with just the right words. I have "listened" when Crystal has wondered why this is happening. I have "listened" in the still of the night...sometimes because of too many pillows in the bed propping up her arms.

Remember when Jesus and His disciples went to the home of Martha? The scriptures say in **Luke 10:39, "*She had a sister called Mary, who sat at the Lord's feet listening to what He said.*"** Now is the time for Crystal...me...and our family to find our place at the feet of Jesus...and to listen.

Many times in the locker room in years past, we asked our players to "listen" to the adjustments that we were making for the upcoming third quarter. Well, now it is Crystal's time to listen. Now it is our time to adjust. As the nurse did for us this afternoon, there is just one more thing to do – "Let's grab hands and pray!" That brought the waterworks out.

As we head into the locker room for halftime, why not grab someone's hand and pray? What adjustments can you make? What are the sounds in your world? Just listen.

I still like the "view from the front."

– **Bill**

Fifteen

Consistently Inconsistent

Friday, August 7

Often that is exactly like my golf game: consistently inconsistent! A good friend asked me this week how I was doing? I used a golf analogy that is all too familiar. You know when you bust that perfect drive, low and with a slight draw, right down the middle of the short grass? You are thinking birdie or par as you prepare for your approach shot. And then you hit it fat...duff...chili dip...more sod than in your yard...standing too close to the ball, after the shot! Now you think about the poor second shot as you hit your third...and fourth. Can't get it off your mind, and that is how one bad swing can ruin a hole and a round. Golf is mostly played between the ears (inside your helmet). Your opponent wants to occupy your mind and put doubt in your thoughts. Then before you know it...your "consistently inconsistent."

Crystal took another trip yesterday to "the plastic!" It was inflation time. Our economy may be in a recession but my wife is feeling the effects of "inflation." Again, see your local breast cancer patient to get more details because it is all new to me too. I just trust that those doctors know what they are doing. (Imagine, people pay good money to go to school to be able to do what they do! Makes my Econ class in college seem like a waste!) This trip tends to make her sore and uncomfortable...which leads to very little sleep for both of us. One more trip and she will be "where she needs to be."

She will go on Monday to see Dr. Fischer again. She has a couple of things to get checked off her pre-treatment list (nothing like a bucket list): get a port put in her collarbone area and have a pet-scan done of her entire body. I don't know when either of these will be done but they will precede the treatment on the 25th. I am sure Dr. Fischer, as he explains our next step, will draw some more pictures on the paper covering the exam table (you know the white paper on the exam tables that make so much noise when you sit on them?). When he told Crystal and I about her having cancer, he took out a blue ink pen and used the paper on the table to show us exactly what she had and where it was and how he would remove it. And praise the Lord HE DID remove it!!

You know I tore that paper off the table and kept it. Crystal looked at me like "What are you doing?". Something told me to take the paper. It is in a safe place in our bedroom. I look forward to the day when I can take that paper and show others saying, "Look what God did for my wife!" Look at what was...and look at what is! Maybe it will help someone else down the road.

You see sometimes as a golfer you can't get a shot out of your mind. You think about it all the time. I was basically telling my friend that life is going on but no matter what we are doing we can't stop thinking about it. It is a constant in our little world. Our children and their activities...but cancer. Work and deadlines to meet...but cancer. Dinner at night and catching up on everyone's day...but cancer. Crystal needing to be a wife and mother...but cancer. That is more like consistently constant!

I am so thankful tonight that our strength comes from someone who is "consistently constant!" There is no inconsistency in Him. *Hebrews 13:8* reminds us that *"Jesus Christ is the same yesterday and today and forever."*

We are the ones who "duff" but He never will let us down. Never a bad swing! You see, just like that paper from the table will one day be used to show others what happened in our lives because of cancer...we should be walking examples of what has happened and IS happening in our lives because of HIM.

Everyday He is constant. Everyday He gives us examples and reasons to share His grace with others. It doesn't have to take being hit with cancer to get us "thinking" about this. Each breath we take...each rain we smell...each smile we see on a child...each call from home...each stranger we pass...each putt we make...we serve an awesome God! He is "consistently consistent!"

So is the "view from the front."

– Bill

Sixteen

Earth, Wind & Fire!

Monday, August 10

Let me paint the picture for you: two **FIRE** trucks, paramedics, police cruiser, lights flashing, sirens roaring, and neighbors watching from their front steps. All Mr. P wanted to do last night was make some cinnamon rolls for the family. You know, a late night snack. Now I know why we have only made them on Sunday mornings all these years. They don't work at night!

He didn't know the oven would flame up!! Get a fire extinguisher! We don't have one!! Run to Mr. Bobby's house Austin! I got one!! Sorry guys but we have it under control. Sorry neighbors, you can ALL go back inside...please STEP AWAY FROM THE YARD! What a night at the Gray house.

You want to forget for a moment about cancer...just open up a can of cinnamon rolls!! You'll forget about cancer fast. You will have a house full of firemen! They will bring the strongest fan you have ever seen (talk about getting rid of dust quickly), literally a **WIND** tunnel. As the scene calmed down and the public servants left the neighborhood you could almost hear my other children (and Billy Joel) singing, "We didn't start the fire!"

We couldn't help but laugh when everyone left. We had the entire family in the house. Briana had missed the excitement but arrived as we were replaying the night. Crystal was in rare form showing how (she claims) I panicked under pressure. Looks like another trip to Home Depot for an extinguisher. The neighbors were probably thinking, "what on **EARTH** can happen next?"

Well, what happened next was... another week started today. We just didn't bake anything for breakfast. We started the day at Dr. Fischer's office. He got out the blue pen again today and was drawing some more pictures. Crystal even said to me as we were leaving, "You're not going to take the paper?". Not this time.

He just showed us how the plastic port will look under her collarbone next Tuesday. She is scheduled for another surgical procedure on Tuesday, August 18th to "put the port in place." (Say that five times.) This will give it one week to settle in her before she starts the third quarter.

We have talked about the adjustments that are sure to come. We have talked about how we are going to attack the opponent. We have talked about how important momentum will be coming out of the locker room. We have talked...we have prayed...we have planned. We are getting her body ready for a long, important second half. I know Team Crystal will "rise up and fight!"

I am amazed at the players who continue to "show up." One of the many things that we enjoyed when we were coaching was to see which player would "show up" on any given night. We continue to see evidence of our God "showing up" on a daily basis. It has been overwhelming at times. It is very humbling for my wife and family.

Team Crystal, we will go into battle with you ANY TIME!

My day ended today much different than last night. There wasn't any "fire and wind" but just one of the sweetest teammates on "earth." A team member came through town and stopped to share...to listen...to encourage...to "show up." He quoted me some scripture in the parking lot. It was from *Psalms 5: 1-3...*

"O Lord, hear me as I pray;
pay attention to my groaning.
Listen to my cry for help, my King and my God,
for I will never pray to anyone but you.
Listen to my voice in the morning, Lord.
Each morning I bring my requests to you and wait expectantly."

His family is playing a tough opponent as well. His family has enough to concentrate on in their own game, but he wanted to "show up." He reminded me how just like a great team we are to wait expectantly! More importantly, just like a child of God, we are to bring our requests to Him...and wait expectantly!

Another... "view from the front."

– Bill

Seventeen

What You Don't Know Won't Hurt You

Thursday, August 13

Ever heard that one before? Sure you have. I'm not sure I totally believe that statement. Some say "Knowledge is Power." Some say "I don't want to know." I don't know...do you?

Tomorrow (Friday), Crystal is scheduled for a couple of tests that we have heard about since our first visit with the oncologist... an echocardiogram and pet scan. The oncologist wants these tests done before the second half begins. This is kind of like taking a player into the training room during half time to make sure he can go for the third quarter. Doc, what do you think...can she play in the second half? We have got to have her ready to go! Get her on the field!!

The first test will determine if her heart is fit for the upcoming treatments. I don't think she has studied for this exam tomorrow, but I feel certain that she will pass the "heart test." I have seen her heart first hand.

I have seen late nights preparing lunches...folding clothes....laying out Easter Sunday surprises...praying for her children...dressed in white at the altar. I have seen her running carpool...taking her own gift cards and buying for her family instead...hurting for someone on the other end of the phone...not saying no...and making us laugh until we cry. Yep, she will blow past this test.

The second test will tell us as best it can whether the cancer has spread to other places in her body. "What you don't know won't hurt you"... I'm not so sure. The doctor says even if it has spread... her treatment would be the same. "What you don't know won't hurt you"...again, I'm not so sure. Doc, convince me that we need to know! Does it reduce our hope? Does it guarantee it isn't there? Is it another statistic to share? Will it "hurt" by knowing?

We go to bed tonight wondering if we need to "know"...but also "knowing"...that she has had her last expansion earlier today. Another night with the discomfort of having seen "inflation" first hand. (How much is that king size bed?) We also know she is, as of tonight, four weeks out of a surgery that will forever change her look in the mirror. (Word is, from a dear friend of ours and a "private" exam, that she is an A+.)

We know also that exactly eight weeks ago our world changed when a doctor looked Crystal in the eye and talked about the sovereignty of God! We know he pulled out that blue ink pen and started drawing. These are some things we know, but is it correct that "what you don't know won't hurt you?"

The Bible says in *Jeremiah 9:24* that if a man wants to boast, let him boast that he *"understands and knows me, that I am the Lord."* When you know this scripture context, you know that it isn't about wisdom or strength or riches...but about knowing Him. I don't know if we will find out anything from tomorrow that we can boast about. I don't know if we will gain wisdom after the tests. I don't know if the news will make Crystal any stronger. I don't know if we will have more change in our pockets after tomorrow. But one thing I do know…if you "don't know Him"…eventually it will hurt you!! This I DO KNOW!

We rest tonight in knowing that God Knows…and that He sees "the view from the front."

– **Bill**

Eighteen

Keeping Watch

Saturday, August 15

"Where is Austin? Why aren't they playing? What did I have for lunch?" These were just some of the questions I got on Friday evening from my wife. You see she had her two tests scheduled yesterday at St. Vincent's. She passed the echocardiogram...I knew she would. Then came the dreaded PET scan. She was to have the PET scan done also at St. Vincent's, but the machine was malfunctioning... broke! She said it was a "sign from the Lord." Something about what you don't know won't hurt you.

Birmingham is a well-known medical community and St. Vincent's provides such great care...but can we not afford more than one PET scan machine? I mean, how much can they possibly be? So, we had to travel across town to another branch of the hospital in order to get the test done (before you ask, she will not have the much anticipated results back until Monday or Tuesday). A guy named Andy (Andy the PET scan guy) called us and directed us to his location. He was even waiting for Crystal in the lobby when I pulled up to the door, apologizing for the inconvenience. Now that is service!

Andy asked us when we arrived, "Where do you guys live?" He said he thought he recognized Crystal's name. You see he goes to church with our neighbors and they have had Crystal on the prayer list for weeks! We had never met Andy before....never been to his church...but he knew our story. He had prayed for my wife! Again, another example of the Lord "placing people" in our path. Broke machine...another hospital across town. Coincidence? I think not. Pretty cool huh!?

Now Crystal had taken a prescription that morning to "take the edge off " of the PET scan procedure. Something about large, loud, metal machines in close proximity to her body doesn't fit well with her nerves. Never knew she had this problem until this cancer thing. Something else I didn't know is that these pills can last for a while...like most of the day. After a late lunch from a long day at the hospitals, we traveled to Austin's football scrimmage out of town.

Now my wife has been to countless football games in her life. She has watched the game as a sister, a parent, and a coach's wife. She knows the game...and she certainly knows where her sons are on the field. While sitting in the stands, the aforementioned questions started coming. "Where is Austin?" ("QB's always line up behind the center baby.") "Why aren't they playing?" ("End of the quarter, taking a break, no time on the clock.") "What did I have for lunch?" ("You ordered chicken and we sat and ate a relaxed meal.") "Taking the edge off " might be an understatement!

We have been reminded in recent days that people are watching. Sometimes watching our actions...our reactions. Sometimes they are watching our children...from a distance...making sure they are ok in this game. Sometimes they are watching those watching us... members of Team Crystal. Always watching.

In **Psalms 121:3** the scriptures remind us that *"He who watches over you will not slumber."* You see, Crystal was at Austin's game but she didn't really know what she was watching. The meds were causing her to basically "look" but not watch. Andy "the pet scan guy" was placed in our path because He who watches over us was not slumbering. Andy was watching for Crystal...God was watching! Our teammates, and so many others, are watching...because God is watching. He is not in slumber.

We know this. We are reminded of this everyday. You are watched over too. *He who watches over us is watching over you as well.*

What an AWESOME promise to grasp hold of! He WATCHES!! Thanks for watching.

That is "the view from the front."

– **Bill**

Nineteen

Go as Can

Tuesday, August 18

Crystal is now the proud owner of the "Power Port!" I don't know really how "proud" she is but she does own one now. It comes with its own wristband and key chain. You might want to rush down to the nearest hospital and pick yours up today...while they last! I just hope the one you get comes easier than the one she picked up today.

I was never in the Army but have been told on many occasions about the "hurry up and wait" motto. We experienced that today. After arriving at the hospital at 9:45 am, she finally went into surgery at 5:00 pm this evening. Nothing to drink...nothing to eat...talk about a late kick-off. It was like a road trip sitting around the hotel ALL day...but worse. "Doc, can we get some relief here?!"

I got to see her in recovery at 6:30 pm and although she didn't look like a rematch with Joe Frazier, (bless her heart) her upper body and arms have been put through the ringer in the last few weeks. Enough of these surgical procedures for a while.

Her left arm is still sore (with some swelling) because of the lymph node removals. Her right arm, we discovered today, is still not recovered from her "seven hour iron drip" while in the hospital last month. Now add to the first surgery a "Power Port" to the upper chest area. Well, some of you know what I am talking about.

We used to classify injured football players in several categories: "Out," "Limited," "Go as Can," and "Full Go." After consulting with our trainer at halftime...my bride would have to be "GO as Can!" You see there is no way she is "out." I saw her today letting two different nurses try and run a drip in her right arm and saying "don't worry, it doesn't hurt." She isn't out! There is no way she is "limited." I saw her battle out of recovery today (thanks to the saltines) and then tell the nurse tonight, "I want to sleep in my bed." She isn't limited!

Since she is on meds tonight and not proofing "my view'," I will mention that the nurses said she was in "rare form" coming out of surgery. That happy juice had her speaking what was on her mind. Suffice it to say, the nurses were eager to share with me what I had missed. Nothing embarrassing. Just my wife holding court! Of course, she remembers none of it.

Now I know she is a long way from being "full go." I see the struggles getting dressed...sleeping through the night...rising from the couch...and picking things up (Crystal, put that down!). No, she isn't "full go"...yet. However, I do know she is "Go as Can." I was always partial to those that were listed "Go as Can." It always gave me an opportunity to see how much they could take...how far they would push themselves...how bad they wanted to get back on the field! She wants to get back on the field. She wants to be in the line-up when the second half starts!

Let me give you a Biblical example of "Go as Can". *Isaiah 40:31* reminds us that *"those who hope in the Lord will renew their strength. They will soar on wings like eagles; they will run and not grow weary, they will walk and not be faint."* Crystal mentioned the other day that she didn't want her cancer to "hinder" the boys this season. She didn't want to "distract" from their football. I told her quickly that she would be a motivation!

Those boys...her boys...will play harder this year than ever before. They will run and not grow weary. She is determined to run and not grow weary. The boys are hoping in the Lord...Crystal is hoping in the Lord...and we have hope in the Lord!

Crystal may be "Go as Can," but it is because of our "hope in the Lord" that she can! The second half is about to start so get your popcorn and get back in your seat. We don't want you to miss one single play. Team Crystal needs you to be a "great cloud of witnesses." We've got the "Power Port." However, we didn't need a port to tell us where "our Power comes from."

From the hospital without a PET scan result yet, to home with a port and a "view from the front."

– Bill

Twenty

Undercover

Thursday, August 20

In the Birmingham area this afternoon, if you were outside, you probably were looking to get "undercover." God was spreading liquid sunshine all over His fertile soil. He reminded us of His power... strong thunder and lightning. He reminded us of His grace...rays of sunshine breaking through dark clouds. He reminded us that sometimes you better have sense enough to get "undercover" during a storm. Come on people! Aren't you glad we have a covering?

Late yesterday afternoon, Crystal got the news from her PET scan. She didn't wait for the call...she made the call. Permission granted by her oncologist to get the news over the phone...no more waiting. Overall, really good news! Her cancer showed up in one additional lymph node, under her left clavicle. Covered up from the doctor's eyes..."undercover." Although this is the fifth lymph node detected with cancer, it shouldn't change her treatment schedule. It is located in an area where the chemo and radiation will be attacking already. Just a lonely, stray cancerous node...once thought safe and "undercover."

What do you do the last few days before you start months of chemo? How do you remember your LBC (life before chemo)? Well, everyone knows the tradition is to have your sister come to town and go shopping for a wig! That is exactly what happened today. Glad I wasn't on the invite list to this party.

I never knew these wigs, or cranium prosthetics as some are called, were this complicated. Do you want real hair or synthetic...one color or showing your roots...long hair or short...same color or different (what about a red-headed Crystal for a while)? Do you want it with or without the comfortable insert that fits to your scalp...attachable bangs or not...special ordered or an in stock model? Moderately priced or second mortgage...will this be an inside wig or worn outside...with or without a cap? Choices, choices, and more choices.

In reality, all we are doing is covering up what I know is going to be a "good looking, lilly white, bald head." A do-rag would be cheaper. We just want to put something on top that will keep her from catching a chill this fall or winter. Something where her head will be "undercover."

I am reminded of a scripture, **Romans 4:7, "Blessed are they whose transgressions are forgiven, whose sins are covered."** As Christians, we can rest in the assurance that our sins are "undercover." They are covered by the blood. Sins of the past...present...and future. A gift of grace...undeserved...often unappreciated...but always forgiven!

Sometimes the fiercest of storms can remind us of being "under God's cover." Remote lymph nodes can't hide from God. They too are "under His cover." LBC or LAC, either way, we have the opportunity and the choice to rest "under His cover." When others see your scalp, it doesn't matter if they see hair or air...dread locks or expressions of shock. What matters is all of it is "under God's cover."

The scriptures give us promise that we are blessed when our sins are "undercover."

God's view is from the top – I still have "the view from the front."
– **Bill**

Twenty-One

Clouds at Hamburger Heaven

Saturday, August 22

I threw a quick question out to the backseat passenger today, "Look at the sky and those beautiful clouds. What are they called?" Bailey responded with "Cumulus!" I had to look next to me at Mr. P to see if she was correct. Of course, she was. Huge, rolling billows of bright white against a Carolina blue sky! Topping the hill on Highway 280 and looking towards Greystone, the three of us were treated to a snapshot of a "picture perfect sky." I didn't want them to miss it.

We were running some errands – new cell phone for Crystal. Her phone got soaked in an empty stadium last night at halftime. You got that snapshot? Scrambling ladies running for cover. ("Are you serious Mr. Verizon man, a one hour wait?")

We decided to attack errand number two – new element for the stove (Mr. P and his C-rolls). But before we could do that...we had to hit Hamburger Heaven, a landmark in the Birmingham area. Saturday afternoon with a couple of your children. Messy burgers... shakes...no appointments to make...blue skies and low humidity.. Good stuff!

I tell you what else is good stuff. Watching your quarterback show "poise" with less than a minute left in the game and down three! Watching your quarterback throw a game winning pass! Knowing that the quarterback you are watching...is your son! Fans screaming... legs tired...clock running...coaches hollering...cheerleaders cheering (and praying)...palms sweating...clock ticking down...referee raising his arms! Poised in the pocket. Might not happen again, but it happened last night. Good stuff.

This is Crystal's last weekend without that poison they call "chemo" running through her body. She will begin her treatments on Tuesday afternoon. Halftime is almost over. The bands have left the field and Team Crystal is coming back out for the second half. She has gotten off her feet...heard the adjustments...seen the trainer...and now has one more piece of coaching advice before she leaves the locker room for the second half. I am leaning over to whisper in her ear, with an arm around her shoulder (just like a quarterback). "Remember, show some poise! When everything seems like it is flying all around you and you can't control it...Be Poised! Look to the clouds for strength and remember...Just Be Poised!"

Webster's dictionary says that to be "poised" is to "hold in a steady position." Not a bad thing to think about but I have something a little better to hang your helmet on in the midst of the storm. It is a verse from our playbook, from *Job 37:16*, *"Do you know how the clouds hang poised, those wonders of Him who is perfect in knowledge?"*

You see the one that puts those cumulus clouds in the sky, the one that can make those same white puffs become dark and grey, the one that seems to have them "poised" in the blue sky...He is perfect in knowledge! He is perfect in knowledge. He knows. He is telling us to "Just Be Poised." He has it in control.

I know Crystal and our family will begin a long six months next Tuesday. A long second half. Team Crystal will have to play hard... but play with "poise." There will be times when it will seem to Crystal like the opposing fans are screaming...like her legs are so tired from playing the game...like the clock is ticking on so slowly...with sweaty palms and people cheering her on...and praying. Steadfastly praying. Praying that we all will look in the end to see our arms raised, not from a referee but from our Team, pointing to the Carolina blue sky. Not to a Hamburger Heaven, but to a God who is "POISED" in Heaven!

Watch her play with "poise" as I watch "the view from the front."
– Bill

Twenty-Two

Waves of Emotion

Tuesday, August 25

Looking back at the last couple of days...

Sunday found us being reminded from so many directions that people really do care. Now, we have felt those prayers specifically over the last few weeks, but it is always good to be reminded. Some reminders came in the form of a text...a note and surprise left in the mailbox...an unannounced knock on the door...a hug from a sweet friend in the church balcony...a hug from a young little girl, that just wanted to "hug Ms. Crystal,"...or a glance with a thumbs up from across the sanctuary.

Even from a deacon behind the pulpit...behind tears. Bailey asked on the way home, "Dad, he was crying for mom wasn't he?" Yeah, I am going to believe that he was....a "wave" of emotions.

Monday the focus was on the next kick-off. That moment right before you leave the locker room to take the field...you can see it in their eyes if your team is ready. If you have ever been in a locker room, then you know what I am talking about. Right at the last minute...their focus is on the task at hand and not the words of a coach. You lose them for just a last brief moment. Let's go coach, let's go!! We had that kind of moment as a family on Monday night.

Waves of emotions.

One particular part of that last moment before leaving the locker room came from a dear friend and her mother. Weeks ago I was asked, "What is Crystal's favorite color?" Kinda reminds me of the old Monty Python scene – "what's your favorite color?" Remember that?

Anyway, little did I know that she wanted to know so that her mother could make Crystal a hand-made, ocean blue crocheted chemo blanket. It took her over two weeks, working at night, to make this special blanket. They surprised Crystal with it Monday night. We are talking about a wave of emotion here! Good stuff... the time and effort...no fanfare, just quietly joining Team Crystal in their own way. Just one of many examples from that day.

Today found us preparing mentally for the second half kick-off! Crystal got more voice mails and texts letting her know that Team Crystal was ready. I heard from Team Crystal supporters as well as several of my coaching friends. One in particular sent me a text about how *Joshua 1:9* reminds us to *"be strong and courageous...not scared...the Lord your God will be with us wherever we go."* I don't know if I have ever received four consecutive texts in a row from the same person, until today. He was so fired up that he was ready to "kick this sucker off and hit this chemo in the mouth!" Talk about a "wave" of emotions – mentally I was running out of the locker room and down to St. Vincent's.

Crystal, of course, can't possibly respond to everyone's encouragement but she reads and hears every one. They are all special because they are from the heart! It touches her heart. It touches my heart to see love expressed...waves of emotions. Thank you all.

OK, this afternoon she got her first treatment in the books. The second half was kicked off about 2:15. She was in the chair for about two and one half hours. Big Red is in her system. The nurse suited up and covered up as she pushed Big Red into my wife's body. Some nasty stuff is working tonight. Do your thing Big Red, do your thing!!

The doctor and nurses told us what to look for over the course of the next few days...days that will become the next few months. To watch Crystal in the chair so many others have sat in with a drip in her "Power Port," it was really a "wave" of emotions for me...as well as her. She was "prayed up" going into that hospital this afternoon! Yet, she still had to climb into that chair. I was proud of her...she looked chemo in the eye. She brought chemo home tonight for the first of many times. Again, we are going to have to play all four quarters of this game.

As I type, she sleeps. As the last few days come to an end, I am reminded of another scripture...one that talks of waves and sleeping in the midst of them. You know the one. It is found in **Matthew 8:24, "Without warning, a furious storm came up on the lake, so that the waves swept over the boat. But Jesus was sleeping."** That is calm assurance.

When we rest in Him, the waves don't bother us. When we rest in Him, there really is no reason for anxiety. Human nature causes us to worry...to be anxious. Jesus wants us to rest...to sleep...in Him.

My prayer tonight is that my wife will feel the comfort of so many prayer warriors protecting our boat from the waves. My prayer is that she will not only rest tonight in her bed, but also in Him. My prayer is that as we play the second half that was started today...we will be reminded that "Jesus was sleeping." It is all in His Control.

Babe, don't be anxious!

You know that is "my view from the front."

– **Bill**

Twenty-Three

Black & White

Saturday, August 29

"Nip it. Nip it in the bud!" "I bet you can even make smoke come out of your ears?!" "It's me, it's me, it's Earnest T." Remember those lines from the Andy Griffith Show (Some of you were worried when I started out this entry with the word "nip")? I love those shows but not as much as one of my friends in Mississippi. I think he knows every line to every show. I am not talking about the later versions of the show when they started filming in color. I am talking about the older ones that were in black and white. Those were the best: simple shows with simple messages...about life! They have stood the test of time because they were simple, and consistent, everyone could relate to life in Mayberry...black and white!

Well our last few days have been mostly "black and white." Nothing really complicated, just simple days, with chemo. Mornings...chemo. Afternoons...chemo. Late nights...chemo. Crystal hit some low spots Thursday and Friday (the steroids in her treatments having worn off). Mostly nausea mixed with a tired body...like the flu but not. Nausea mixed with a bad taste that will not go away. Mostly nausea mixed with problems at the other end. Get the picture? She had a glow to her but it was redness from the steroids, not the glow of a pregnant women...been there, not doing that!

Her tastes have been altered. Food doesn't taste the same, although cravings for potato soup and mashed potatoes have surfaced. She needs to continue to hydrate with water, however, everything feels like it will come right back up. Toughest part of coaching so far this half has been the water. Not much appetite...not much energy...not much fun.

Although her second half just started, those of you who have played this opponent before, know exactly what we are experiencing and what is coming later in the second half. Your insights have been valuable. So after getting treatment number one on Tuesday and just having a simple "chemo life,"...just black and white for a few days.... she was able to find some color in her world. Our family was able to experience some color in our world. Black and white days are ok in Mayberry but not in Hoover.

Color came in the form of "gratefulness." Crystal talked this week about how overwhelming everything has been and all the kindness that has been shown. She made the statement, "How can I ever say thank you to all these people?" I told her, "The best way to thank everyone is to keep fighting this thing and to put yourself in a position to assist the next person who walks where you are walking. People will know how much they have meant to you." I hope each of you know!

Color came in the form of pink ribbons. As you can imagine, pink is becoming a popular color at our house. On Friday night, Crystal insisted on going to Austin's game...in bed at 4:00 pm and in the stadium at 6:30 pm. She was going...maybe not for long...but she was going. Well, she went and stayed! She thanked the girls at the school for making the gift basket and getting the t-shirts done in her honor. Pink ribbons of color and love, just wanting to join the team.

Color also came last night in the form of a "kiss." You have to know my boys to understand the significance of this kiss. After coming off the field for pre-game warm-ups, Austin veered from the locker room and came over to his mom sitting in the Jeep. Sweaty, stinky, full uniform, focused on the opponent....but focused also enough to thank Crystal for coming and to kiss her on the cheek. If you looked close enough at the friends gathered around...you probably saw a few watery eyes! The game had just become the icing on the cake.

I was also reminded this week about the color red. Our week started out focused on "Big Red" in Crystal's veins. That awful, smelly poison that is part of "nipping this cancer in the bud." Rather black and white why they do it...hit cancer in the mouth right off the bat!

However, the later part of the week I was reminded of the color "red" in the Red Sea. I was reminded that God had not placed His children in that position to cause them harm. He had not forgotten them. He knew (and knows) what He is doing.

In *Hebrews 11:29*, it starts by saying *"By faith the people passed through the Red Sea as on dry land..."* Did you get that? By *FAITH* the people passed through. We are faithfully believing that Crystal has better days next week. We are faithfully believing that people are praying daily for her health (imagine how bad she would have felt this week had it not been for prayer!) We are faithfully believing that our children are growing so much from this journey that our family is on. We are faithfully believing that just like God's people in the Old

Testament...He has not brought us to cancer without a plan to make it to the other side. I have faith when I watch a black and white episode of Andy Griffith that at the conclusion, I will be fulfilled. I also have faith that the "colors of God's plan" will continue to show up in our chemo world.

I am able to see those colors because I have "a view from the front!"

– Bill

Twenty-Four

Play Doh

Wednesday, September 2

Do they still make that stuff? Can you still remember it between your hands? I used to make a snake. Easy to do, just roll it against a hard surface...but not the carpet. You would get in some big time trouble if you did two things with Play Doh: leave it out of the container (becomes hard as a rock) or get it in the carpet. Never to come out.

You also better not mix it together if you didn't want it to forever change colors. Play Doh. I am glad my kids weren't hooked on that stuff. Crystal reminded me that our kids played with it but I was always at practice. She would use wax paper to keep the mess clean. I just wasn't around to see (I missed a few more things I am sure). Our carpet may have had stains but they weren't from Play Doh.

You see, when something is not used as it was intended...it can become hard and forever changed. Hard is not good when soft is preferred. Forever changed can't go back.

Crystal has had a better last three days. She still feels the effects of her first treatment in her body, but the nausea is gone for the time being. Thank you Lord! Her medicine, her chemo, is being used as it was intended...but it is still hard.

This particular cycle that she is on is powerful...which is why she only goes every other week for the first eight weeks. The chemo attacks all the fast developing cells in her body. That is why next week, about Wednesday or Thursday, her hair will let go (Who Loves You Baby). Hair grows fast so it gets attacked. That is why her stomach seems to always be upset. The cells in the walls of our intestines grow fast...chemo attacking. But hey, it is still better than the low point of last week. Used correctly, but still hard on the body.

Crystal made the statement the other day, "I don't think I am going back for round two." Say what?! That thought didn't last long but it did stop me in my tracks. She made a wry smile. I know there was some truth to what was said, but not enough to keep her out of the chair next week. I know getting stuff out of the carpet is hard but it pales in comparison to making that trip next Tuesday back to the cancer center.

Food isn't tasting the same these days for her which leads to not much appetite. Every now and then she will find something she likes. Taste buds and cells in the mouth grow fast. Get the picture? Her body is mixed with Big Red and it seems like it will never be the same...like the color has changed forever...but I know different. Although the third quarter just got started, she will get to the final play in due time. Patience.

Today, we were reminded of how God not only has us in the palm of His hand but also has treated us like 'Play Doh'. Crystal was given a special cross today that someone held in their hand...and now she can hold in hers. It brought a scripture to mind. In *Isaiah 64:8* we find these words, ***"Yet, O Lord, you are our Father. We are the clay, you are the potter; we are all the work of your hand."*** I hope that is as comforting to you today as it is for Crystal and I.

He has formed each of us, long ago. He knew the soft would become hard. He knew the stomach would be upset. He knew the cells would be attacked. He knew the hair would let go. He knew the color would be mixed...He ordained it all.

In a world where surgeons can do superb work on the body...it doesn't compare to what the Potter did to His clay. He isn't worried about stains...the blood can wash those away. He wants to soften our hard hearts. He doesn't want His workmanship covered up in hair. We are all the work of His hand.

As He was forming my wife, He had a clear view of the future. I just have "a view from the front."

– Bill

Twenty-Five

A Weekend of Firsts

Monday, September 7

You couldn't drive anywhere this weekend without seeing the colors. In the stores and restaurants...they were everywhere. At school (and even from the Governor himself who declared last Friday as a day to show your colors) many would say the weekend they have been waiting for all year – college football is here! The first weekend of games across the country. A weekend of firsts: first wins, first losses, and first punches thrown (the guy from Oregon didn't tell the guy from Boise to "duck"). A weekend of firsts. Life is good on the first fall Saturday in September...football is here.

I spent Sunday afternoon watching my college roommate's son play his first college football game. I am getting old. He is getting old. A lot of "grey" in the seats, some on my head and some on his face. His son scored his first ever college touchdown (to win the game no less). First time to celebrate. First time to call home to his mom with excitement in the voice. I am sure there will be many more. Glad my friend gave me a chance to experience it with him. Cancer and football seem to give us reasons to reunite old friendships. A Sunday of firsts.

This weekend we saw another first...the first strands of hair on the pillow and the floor. Reality is setting in that we will soon see a new look for the first time. The texture is different than it used to be... Big Red does that. With every shower, Crystal finds more on the floor. We are scheduling a family "shave night." Talk about getting predictions right. Those people at the cancer center know...fourteen days out and you better get ready. Well...you never really get ready!

Today, we are having another first. We are preparing for our first return trip to the chair tomorrow. This one is much different than the first trip. It is one thing to think, it is another thing to know. This time she knows what to expect. Each scenario has its on degree of difficulty. You know the old question about "would you rather know the future or not?" Well Crystal knows.

The first five minutes of the second half are very important in a football game. A lot of times a team will come out and show some different looks that they were saving for the second half. They are either trying to keep or change the momentum. Momentum is very important in the game of football...and the game of life. You have to have a team that can focus on playing "one play at a time." You can't look ahead and you certainly can't look behind!

In the game of football, there are always about four or five plays that determine the outcome...that determine when momentum is shifted. You saw it this weekend in any game you watched...game changing plays. Just a few. If we knew when they were coming we could prepare...but we don't. Each next play could be "the play" that changes the game. So, you just play the next play...one play at a time.

Crystal will get up in the morning and play the next play. She may have a little less hair. She may not like the results of the day, but she will play the next play anyway. We are early in the second half and momentum is very important. Each trip to the chair could be the trip...the play...that changes her momentum against this cancer. Big Red, we are coming back for round two and we are going to look you right in the eye...and not duck!!

We do all this because of the greatest of firsts, the only first that matters, the first of firsts!! ***Revelation 1:8*** reminds my wife and family today that a weekend of small firsts doesn't stand up to the author of firsts. The scripture says this, *"I am the Alpha and the Omega," says the Lord God, "who is, and who was, and who is to come, THE ALMIGHTY."* That, my friend, is a first that will color you with comfort. A first that will punch fear in the gut. A first that will give you momentum to make it. A first that will make your hair stand on end...if you have hair!!

This may be the first entry in a few days, but it is still "my view from the front."

– Bill

Twenty-Six

What Else...Hair!

Wednesday, September 9

You don't find much of it in the board room. I guess age and maturity takes care of it. You see less from the front and more of the lighter shade on top. Distinguished looks seem to make people listen...when around a table with ties. Business is business...not much flowing in the wind inside.

The helmet makes it difficult to have much either, unless you wear the black and gold of Pittsburg...or you play in Canada and your name is Hill. He was the first I have ever coached that the length was not a factor in my eyes. I said often that as long as he played "lights out" (and he did), and was a gentleman off the field (and he is), then it could grow down to his waist. Just keep making plays and staying humble. Don't know if they have the same rules in Canada, but it is covering up part of his number...still growing... dread locks (Mr. P wants some!).

You see all colors on the street. You can even buy color in a box, or pay a fortune to let someone else do it. If you are a Hollywood icon, some will even pay money for a few in a Ziploc bag...on EBay. When we were younger, it was short. As we grew older, it became long. One has it wavy and another has it straight. Some like it laying flat...and others have it stiff with gel!

Throughout the scriptures it is mentioned. Two characters come to my mind: Samson and Absalom. The first had strength in his...but she wouldn't stop trying to find the source. The second got his hung up in the trees while riding a mule in the woods...being chased...he was killed. Great stories. Stay away from those that ask too many questions...and low hanging limbs!

We find it mentioned in so many places. In Leviticus it is mentioned with different colors and associated with sores and being clean and unclean. In Numbers, it is about dedication and sacrifice. In Proverbs the grey means splendor of the old...I really like that one!! John reminds us that Mary wiped Jesus' feet with hers...mixed with tears...awesome picture!

Last night we had a family moment in the kitchen. Crystal's was beginning to come out on its own…pillow...sink...shower...brush. It was time to have a moment. I don't know if any of our family has ever had a prayer before a cut...but we did last night. We just wanted to make sure we were on the same page...like a good team.

Everyone participated. Some wanted a Mohawk. Some didn't want to hurt her. It was the next step...the next play in the second half. And you know what? There were no tears! Pictures captured a moment not many get to have with their children...and son-in-law. Line up guys. We are all getting a turn, but no Ziploc bags (Crystal didn't want the clippers touching anyone else either...she wants to be able to see ours).

As I watched...and later looked...I couldn't help but think of a couple of other verses of scripture. I started to quote her the verse from Song of Solomon where it talks about *"your hair is like a flock of goats descending from Mount Gilead."* Something told me that she wouldn't find that very encouraging! I don't think a woman on chemo wants to be compared to goats coming out of the mountains.

The other verse however, is a great reminder to her and to us.

Not the one in Judges where it says *"the hair on his head began to grow again after it had been shaved."* We already know that is going to happen, although it will be next year sometime. The one I like is from *1 Peter 3:3, "Beauty shouldn't come from outward adornment such as braided hair."* I know it may be a little out of context...but it still fits the season.

Crystal has several options now when she leaves the house. She found a really good looking wig. She has several wraps or "do-rags." Or she can just go 'G.I. Jane or G.I. Crystal'! But you know what? It doesn't matter to me. Last night she showed she can play this Game...against any opponent! Her beauty is not determined by her locks of hair...but by her eyes! They are the mirror to her soul...a reflection of her spirit. A fighter who wants to be tender...one who still makes an awesome picture!

Yes...I still like "my view from the front!"

– Bill

Twenty-Seven

More of the Same...

Monday, September 14

"The Israelites ate mana forty years…" (Exodus 16:35).

Remember the movie Groundhog Day? It was based on the premise that everyday Bill Murray woke up...it was the same day. He saw the same people, heard the same noise, went to the same places... until. Until he figured out that he could make each day different! He could change the course of the events around him...if he so desired. He might even have a chance to get the girl in the end. I don't know that I would recommend renting the movie...unless you wanted to do something "different" one weekend.

I know it has been a few days since I journaled...but that has been for two reasons. One reason is the author has been a little under the weather (aren't we all literally under the weather?). However, a large nurse with a needle in her hand and your pants pulled down will make you get well quick!! The other reason for not writing is that around here...it has been a little like 'Groundhog Day'.

Now, we haven't seen a furry critter running around dodging his shadow, but Crystal has basically had the same feeling, the same bad taste in her mouth, the same nausea, the same lack of energy, and the same hair-do for the last several days. Treatment number two was last Tuesday and she is just now coming out of the haze. She had a couple of steroids to take home this time to help with some of the side effects.

So, she is ready for her "good week." Her hair-do is changing a little. Anyplace where her head rubs against something – her pillow, the couch, her bandanna – she finds a white spot. No tan on that head! I would think in the next few days we will have another party in the kitchen...this time with a razor. One good thing is that she can get dressed as fast as anybody now...no time spent on the hair!

Football is the toughest of sports for many reasons. One main reason is all the monotonous practice that you must endure for one chance a week to put on those silks and turn on the lights. Practicing the same things over and over. Every Monday is the same. Every Tuesday is the same. And on and on. Yet, those that can endure, especially in a tough game...in the second half...can fall back on all the preparation that went into a game plan. They then can execute without thinking! They can raise their heads with confidence that they have prepared!

It has been 60 days since Crystal's surgery...two months. Sometimes it seems longer. It has been 20 days since her first chemo Treatment. Time doesn't fly when you aren't having fun. She can't see the finish line, the end of the fourth quarter, but it is out there. She just has to keep working...keep pressing on. Her time will come. Every day doesn't have to be the same. She is learning that her attitude is going to play a big role in this victory. Of course the sickness gets old. But keep looking up...with confidence.

In *Exodus 34:28*, Moses was with the Lord for 40 days and 40 nights without eating or drinking water. Yet, after enduring, he brought down the Ten Commandments. He was with God!

In *Mark 1:13*, Jesus was in the desert for 40 days being tempted by Satan. He endured and Satan was defeated. God was with Him!

Although the Israelites ate mana for 40 years, it wasn't because God was not there. He was! The mana came from Heaven! He opened up the skies to provide all they needed. He is still in the business of providing us with all we need. It is just too often that we think we can do it on our own...that we have all the answers.

During the period of 40 days between Crystal's surgery and when she had her first chemo treatment, we prayed that God would provide! We prayed that He would provide Crystal with healing...strength... patience...peace...strong faith...a sense of humor...a spirit of no fear... hope. She has been prayed up by so many people in so many parts of the world, literally (just read the places on the guestbook). We are so thankful for that. During these last 20 days we can understand why. This chemo is tuff !!

So, we are looking to the skies...looking to heaven...knowing where our strength comes from. Team Crystal is playing this second half with a head held high...with confidence...looking for God to provide!

Looking up...but still "the view from the front."
– Bill

Twenty-Eight

Sinks, Saints, Sore Throats and Surprises

Friday, September 18

Did you hear the gasp earlier this week? Did your world stop in its tracks? Better yet, did the world continue to spin...as usual? What am I talking about? My wife left the house one day this week without cleaning out the dishwasher and with dirty dishes in the sink! We are all pitching in to do dishes now, but for some reason a few didn't get done the night before. And when spotted the next morning...she didn't care! There can only be one explanation. Crystal was sick. And for that day, that morning, the dishes didn't matter.

We all have our lists, our things to do, things that we want done. Things that cause us not to rest until they have been checked off. I can count on one hand (no, really one finger) how many times she hasn't cared about the dishes in our marriage. There is nothing wrong with a clean sink....unless your energy level is so low that it is no longer a priority. It just isn't worth it!

Now before you think that they are stacked up like a restaurant... and come running down the street with a clothe...don't. Our kitchen would be in the top ten in cleanliness. However, this speaks to how rough the "good week" was this past week. Some things...at least for a morning...just weren't nearly as important.

Our family was reminded this week that the world is full of "saints"..we just need to look closer....and appreciate their presence. I joined a group of old friends, and players, to celebrate the life of one precious saint on Tuesday. Always smiling in the stands...always spreading the gospel...always an encourager...a true saint. I had the privilege to coach her son. She had the privilege to leave a wonderful testimony...and family. How many times has someone driven almost an hour...at six o'clock in the morning....just to pray with you? Her husband did....and I will never forget that day.

And there are so many days that Crystal will not forget because of all the "saints" that have crossed our paths these last few months. It was said over dinner tonight, "I have never seen an outpouring of love by so many for one family in all my life." We haven't either. Not necessarily a New Orleans fan...but I sure love the saints!

Chemo has caused her throat to become tender, like a severe strep. There is a medical term for it but let's just say it is a side effect of Big Red. Because of this, food is not attractive and liquids don't go down easy...both of which she needs consistently. Therefore, she has lost some weight. The chemo diet. Magic Mouthwash is on the cabinet, but hard to put in the throat. The head may be smooth...but the throat is not!

Crystal's birthday was this past week. Four days younger than me. Talk about robbing the cradle! Although we have known for a long time her birthday was coming...we didn't know it would be one for the books. Although on her birthday she didn't feel good enough to celebrate...there would be a tomorrow.

She had a surprise when a knock on the door brought her brother, Steve, for a surprise visit (I can keep a secret). She got to see the surprise look on her parent's face also, when they saw her "new look" for the first time (a visit they have been wanting to make as well). She even found out that shopping for hats...can produce a very good looking image...surprise, surprise!! She now owns three!

This "off week" was supposed to be a "feel good" week. Well, it didn't quite live up to the expectations...physically. However, the week exceeded expectations in reminding our family that we serve an awesome God. From six year olds to shopping...there were numerous opportunities for us to Praise the Lord. Despite the surroundings and the conditions and the "stuff " that life throws our way, we can be reminded of what is said in ***Psalms 103:11: "Bless the Lord, O my soul; and all that is within me, Bless His Holy Name!"***

Looking at a beautiful smile....and a light blue hat...with "my view from the front."

– Bill

Twenty-Nine

Hooked Up & Hanging Out

Wednesday, September 23

The room needs paint. Some windows wouldn't hurt either. Who was the person that said "flat tan" would look good on a hospital wall? I mean, come on! A picture or two would also be a nice touch. I know we can't do too much about the furniture. The chairs don't look like something in your den...but they do the job. And you can forget carpet...hard floors...hard looks. Doesn't sound like a place you want to visit does it? Well, neither does Crystal. However, she was there yesterday getting treatment number three!

When I walked around the corner to check and see how she was, I found her "hooked up and hanging out!" The patients have a port that gets "hooked up" with the chemo and the tubes "hang out" about twelve inches from their body. This particular room only has four chemo chairs and each one had a patient. There were three women and one man this time. Poor fellow....has to get a treatment...and listen to three chemo charged ladies for several hours. Crystal said he slept most of the time!

Each patient had something in common: chemo flowing thru their port. However, each patient was different. One lady, for instance, would have a six hour session (Crystal's session lasted about three hours total). One may be on the last of her cycle... while another may be getting her first dose. Yet, each was placing confidence in the fact that in order to heal the body...they had to tear it down. The chemo doesn't know what is or is not cancer. So, it just attacks...and attacks...and attacks.

Crystal is feeling the "side effects" of the chemo quicker with each treatment. By the time Tuesday afternoon came yesterday she was ready to settle somewhere for the evening. This is a lot faster than her first time when she didn't feel anything until the next day. The body must be collecting more and more of "the stuff." We were reminded again that "these first four will be tough." As always, our prayer is that she will get over the rough days quicker as well, and have a "good week" on this cycle. Good weeks make everyone feel better.

So, there she was comparing hats...scarves...and wigs (I told you the guy was sleeping). They were comparing side effects as well. Any tips on this bad taste in my mouth...What about foods, does anything taste good to you...What are you doing for nausea? It was a good opportunity to gather information from others that are playing the same opponent. A lot like watching and exchanging game film in football. I just wish they had a prettier room with some pictures or windows.

Crystal isn't the only one in the family who is "hooked up and hanging out." Briana has started a running club at Samford. They meet once a week at night. Late night (do college students do anything early?)...and run for a cause. They run...for Crystal. The group has about thirty members, both guys and girls, with about twenty that show up to run on any given week.

They are training to run in next month's Race for the Cure in Birmingham. Team Crystal will be well represented on Saturday, October 10th. When asked what color t-shirts to get, the guys said they wanted pink of course. Pink and Proud!! It has really made her mom proud. Each of our children are handling this in their own way. This is one way Briana is dealing with her mom's cancer.

However, there is one little problem that comes with this running group. We are not sure what needs to go on the back of the shirts. One suggestion is "Save the Ta-Tas!" Another is... "Run for the Hills!" (I think I will stop there). I am sure they will get a consensus on something. It doesn't hurt to put a smile on someone when you pass them in a 5k run.

A more conservative phrase for the back of a shirt...or the front of a fridge...or to hide in your heart, is found in **Hebrews 12:1b**. It says, *"...and let us run with perseverance the race marked out for us."* Just like a football game develops over the course of four quarters, Crystal's contest, her race, is developing with each treatment. She has to continue to persevere because the end justifies the means. This is the race that has been set out for her to travel.

Briana's group is "hooked up and hanging out" in order to do what they can for Crystal and her fight. The new friends that Crystal is meeting at the hospital are "hooked up and hanging out" for one another each time they go into that awful looking room. Our family continues to praise the Lord for those of you who are "hooked up and hanging out" because of this website...and because of your love and care for Crystal and our family.

Working to get into shape...and looking forward to wearing pink...that is "my view from the front."

    – **Bill**

Thirty

Protect the Rock!

Tuesday, September 29

When that pigskin gets loose...one side cheers...and the other side kicks and screams. When that "brown, oblong object" hits the turf...one thing is certain...the stadium is going to fill with emotion! Half good, and half bad. Half excited, and half mad. All eyes are on the "object of affection"...the rock. Any player that carries it knows it needs to be protected! Fumbles have made some coaches start drinking...or selling insurance...or working at a bank!

If you live in our neck of the woods, this fall you have seen teams all around that have had to concentrate on ball security...because it has rained practically every weekend. Football in the rain...always exciting. Plays can still be made but the teams that make them are the ones that "protect the rock." They are the ones that realize that the rain falls on both sides of the stadium. Use it to your advantage!

Last Thursday, watching Austin's game...muddy field. I mean a stinking, muddy field (the kind where short people disappear). The opposing coach caught my attention. He wasn't making excuses. He was determined to keep his focus.

He came out in his nice white long sleeve shirt, with tie, with nice slacks...but with no shoes!! His shoes kept coming off, getting "sucked into the mud." He overcame the situation...roll up your slacks and take 'em off...but keep coaching. Austin's team won the game big, but that coach got my attention. He was teaching his kids a lesson...do what you have to do.

On Saturday, the boys and I went to Auburn to see Bailey perform at halftime of the Ball State game, in the rain, on a wet field, and with about 1,199 other cheerleaders. They looked like ants... wet ants... colorful wet ants...especially when they decided half way thru the routine to change ends of the field...quickly. I was praying Bailey wouldn't fall down or get run over during the exchange, but she handled it like a pro. She didn't let a wet field cause her to lose her balance...or concentration (wonder where she got that athletic ability?). She did what she had to do!

So did the boys. Because Crystal was not having a great weekend, she missed both of these events plus half of Mr. P's game on Friday (she could only handle the first half...even though she had on a nice white hat!). They didn't let that stop them from doing what they had to do. A lot of that these days.

They not only played their games...and won...but got up on Saturday and represented the family in Auburn. In the rain...making a memory (at least that is what they heard from me as we drove down in the down pour). This is a day that your little sister will always remember....the day you guys sat in the rain for her! Now quit complaining and act like your having fun!

So, what about Crystal? After several days of not feeling well, she went to the hospital today for some fluids....a big bag of fluids.

Dehydration...because of a poor appetite, because of nausea, and because of the effects of treatment number three with Big Red (have I told you lately that this stuff is tough on the body?)! Thank the Lord for fluids from a bag! In that hospital room today it was like "rain from heaven." Crystal came home feeling, at least for tonight, so much better.

Psalms 72:6 says, "He will be like rain falling on a mown field, like showers watering the earth." You know the look of a field...maybe a football field...which has just been rained on? You know how it shines in the stadium lights? A thing of beauty! Although it has been raining on Team Crystal during these last few days...plays have still been made. Plays that we will talk about for weeks to come...just like that coach with mud between his toes.

Some recent "big plays" have been: trash cans being put back into place from the street...neighbors showing up at games to replace Crystal...prayers from co-workers in an e-mail...phone calls...a map of the United States that shows where people are praying for Crystal..food, food and still more food...cards of encouragement... packages at the door...and even muffins and Lucy movies! The rain has not stopped Team Crystal's players from making plays. They are doing what they want to do!

Crystal's face tonight was like that shiny, damp field under the lights. Her body had been blessed with some liquids...liquids hanging from "above." Even though her field may be wet and muddy, she is going to continue to do what needs to be done. That may not mean she can do everything she wants to...but that is why she has teammates. We are going to protect "the rock...our object of affection!"

The rain does indeed fall on both sides of the stadium. I am glad we are resting tonight in knowing who brings the rain.

I want to know, "Have you ever seen the rain?". Damp...but "my view from the front."

  – **Bill**

Thirty-One

Chinese Words and Toothless Sounds

Tuesday, October 6

This past Friday found me and a friend going to the south Alabama town of Monroeville to watch Austin play football. After a two and a half hour ride, we stopped at a convenience store to ask for directions to a local eatery, some place that was unique for this town. Who would have thought that behind the counter I would find someone who only spoke fluent Chinese...in Monroeville?! Getting directions to anywhere became a major problem (I needed my next door neighbors, young girls Katy Bi and Cally, to translate!). Sounds...

There was one customer in the store at the time who volunteered to help us. However, there was a problem...the customer was a lady who was toothless. Have you ever gotten directions from a toothless lady telling you the only place to eat is the Huddle House? Is there anyone in Monroeville who we can understand? Well we found our own way to an outstanding all-u-can-eat catfish place, Dave's Catfish House...a popular spot, sitting right next to the Huddle House. Dave's motto on his t-shirts is: Promote Catfish...Run Over a Chicken! You can't make this up! Sounds...

If you had been at Austin's game, you would have heard the sounds from the home stands in the second half...getting louder with each first down. The small school from down south won this contest. Partying at Dave's...not many sounds heading north back to Birmingham. Sounds...

Mr. P's game had the same outcome for the Gray family. The blue and white behind his bench had a lot to shout about in the first half ! The side wearing black made the most noise in the end. Have you noticed, the higher the score....the more noise you hear? Football has a way of doing that on a Friday night...not a lot of sounds coming from our house by night's end. Sounds...

Crystal had her fourth and final "Big Red" treatment today...did you hear the sound? She didn't want to climb back into the chair, but she was glad to get out when she was done. Did you hear the sound? She is having a good evening but knows when the sun comes up, her body will begin to feel the poison. Still, did you hear the sound?

There were several sounds today that we heard....and you may have heard also. The click of the tube being taken out of her port... knowing that the red fluid will flow no more into her body...a wonderful sound The doctor telling her today that her blood work looks good and after this treatment the next round will be easier on her body...a welcome sound! Messages left on the answering machine letting her know, as if she didn't, that she was prayed up today while in the chair...sweet sounds!

Our journey last Friday took us to parts unknown and we heard sounds we didn't understand. Remember Saul on the Damascus road that changed his life? Remember his team that traveled with him and their response to the sound? *Acts 9:7* tells us, *"The men traveling with Saul stood there speechless; they heard the sound but did not see anyone."* The sound was that of Jesus speaking...a sound that changed Saul forever!

Dave's Catfish was good, but it won't change my life. I am also sure I will hear the sound of directions again one day. Losing football games hurt, but only for a short time...until the sounds of winning come back. The sounds Crystal heard today lifted her spirits and will help her sleep well tonight...until the nausea returns. However, the sound that resonates forever in our hearts, is the sound of Jesus being allowed to come in and change our lives...forever. That's a sound that needs no translation...a sound that has teeth!!

Thanks for listening to the sounds of "my view from the front."

– **Bill**

Thirty-Two

TIME OUT!

Wednesday, October 14

You get three per half. Use them, cause you can't carry them over to the next half...or to the next game. Sometimes...you have to stop momentum. Sometimes...you have to make sure everyone is on the same page. Sometimes...you aren't lined up correctly. Sometimes... you don't have enough players...or too many...or the wrong personnel. Sometimes...you have to make a point with your team! Can you give me a time out!

That is what happened last Saturday morning. A rainy...wet... early...wonderfully pink Saturday morning. After getting to bed late Friday night because of recapping the football games the boys played (Crystal stayed home, not feeling well), it was tough for everyone to get up and head to downtown Birmingham for the Race for the Cure...especially hard for Crystal. Although she didn't have to do her hair, it is still tough for her to get up and out in the early morning. But she was motivated on this day...

Briana had worked very hard to organize a group of friends from

Samford to run for Team Crystal. Everyone had matching pink shirts, wet hair, smiles on their faces, love in their hearts, and an eagerness to run for a lady some had never met! To RUN FOR THE HILLS!! That was reason enough for anybody to get up and out on this Saturday. But there was more.

All of our kids were involved as well. Briana and Payton ran the 5k. Brittany and Bailey walked and fellowshipped their way around the course. Austin (after playing a tough game the night before) and I stayed with Crystal to watch and cheer. (You have to have a good support team.) Friends from our church, our Sunday school class, and neighbors across the street ran and walked for Crystal and others...14,000 runners and walkers in all. Everyone on the same page.

Before this past Saturday, many in our family had never thought about participating in this annual affair...but that was before. That was before we "felt the word cancer." That was before we saw first hand the "sea of pink." That was before the lady that we had never seen before ran up to Crystal and stopped and pointed at her...and said, "Today, I am running for YOU!" That was before this past Saturday...before as a family...we took a TIME OUT!

Crystal has just finished her four treatments of "Big Red." She will begin next Tuesday with a different chemo treatment, once a week for twelve straight weeks, phase two you might call it. It was a good time to call a "time out." A time to get everyone together and to be reminded that she is not in this alone. A time to see so many who have fought this same fight and won. A time to be reminded that God is in control...and our family is blessed! It was a good time for our family to experience a "time out" in this game. To just stop... and enjoy the morning.

Joshua 10: 13b-14 is a great couple of verses. This came to mind during her initial surgery, and comes to mind again today. Listen to what they say, *"...the sun stopped in the middle of the sky and delayed going down about a full day. There has never been a day like it before or since, a day when the Lord listened to a man. Surely the Lord was fighting for Israel."*

You know, even though the rain was falling, last Saturday seemed like the "sun stopped in the middle of the sky." There were too many "things" that happened in and around that run in downtown Birmingham that just weren't coincidence. It was as if the "Lord was listening to a man"...many men...and women...in pink.

I will share some of those "things" that happened in the next entry.

For now, with a little "time out" in between...that is "my view from the front."

– Bill

Thirty-Three

Waiting on My Eggs

Tuesday, October 20

Following the "Race for the Cure" a couple of Saturdays ago, the entire family went to The Ranch House – a popular restaurant in Vestavia. Well, the entire family didn't go. Justin had to work that day. We missed him.

As always, the place was packed and people were in line waiting. Breakfast until noon will do that on a Saturday. People..."waiting on eggs!"

Ever been in a crowded eatery...waiting on your name to be called? Thinking about leaving and going somewhere less crowded...and quicker? But what if our name is called next? It is the same way in a football game...the next play might be the one! In baseball, the next pitch could turn the game! I have a friend who declares every time the phone rings, "That could be THE CALL! It just takes ONE!" We decided to keep waiting that Saturday morning..."waiting on those eggs!"

We drew the attention of everyone inside when we all walked in with our pink "Team Crystal" shirts! After a few minutes of standing,

Crystal was able to sit on a bench, next to a lady she didn't know. It was a lady who was a breast cancer survivor...for many years...who encouraged Crystal to "keep the faith"...all while "waiting on her eggs!"

That morning there were two different ladies that sat next to Crystal and shared their stories...ladies she had never seen before. Ladies who had a fondness for the color pink...and the promise of a cure! I am one to believe that those women weren't there by accident or coincidence. They were there for a purpose...and not just to "wait on their eggs!"

I shared this with my Sunday Bible study class and one of my friends spoke up that he also had a story from that Saturday morning. He too had gone to The Ranch House that day, however, he went earlier in the morning. When he saw someone he knew already eating in the restaurant, the man asked my friend "where his wife was today?" My friend said that his wife was "running in the Race for the Cure today." Then, the person...who we don't know... asked my friend, "Is she running for Crystal Gray today? We have her name on our prayer list at church and have been praying for her for weeks!" My friend just thought...he was going to be "waiting on his eggs!"

You know the verse that talks about waiting patiently? *In Psalms 40:1, we find... "I waited patiently for the Lord; He turned to me and heard my cry."* You never know what we might be taught...when we wait...patiently.

Over-medium has always been my favorite. The kids are partial to scrambled...with some bacon mixed in. Crystal likes to add some cheese, melted of course. I can even enjoy one boiled with some salt in the middle of the day.

We have eaten them hundreds of times in our lives. But you know, after that Saturday morning...in a crowded breakfast spot...I will always remember the way God spoke to my wife...and to our family in pink. He spoke through people we did not know...while "waiting on my eggs!"

On that day, that was "My view from the front."

– **Bill**

Thirty-Four

All Alone in a Crowded Room

Tuesday, October 20

(the second entry in the same day...don't get used to it...just a long day at the hospital)

In the movie *Pursuit of Happyness*, the final scene has Will Smith's character walking down a street in San Francisco with his son. His son is asking him a knock-knock joke. It went like this, "Knock knock." "Who's there?" "Nobody." Nobody Who?" Then silence. The son said nothing. Finally Will Smith laughed, "Oh, I get it, nobody there!"

Have you ever had times in your life when no one seemed to be there? Ever thrown an interception? Booted a ground ball? Made a bad loan? Had too many days left in the month? Failed a test? Taken a stand against the majority? Gotten the call you feared? Turned the lights out with cancer in your body? We all have in some form or another. We have had the feeling like we were "all alone in a crowded room!" Regardless of what was said...or who was there... we were by ourselves. Or at least that is how it seemed at the time.

Today, Crystal began her second phase of chemo. She began taking Taxol, once a week for the next twelve weeks. Did you know Taxol is from a plant, a plant alkaloid? It is made from the bark of the Pacific Yew tree (if it isn't a magnolia, an oak or a southern pine, I don't know much about it. Plant alkaloids are cell-cycle specific, which means they attack the cells during various phases of divisions. The only problem is they don't know which cells are cancer and which are not...so they attack all the cells that are dividing. Am I keeping you on your 'chemo toes' with this cancer lesson? That is why the throat hurts...the hair lets go...the eyelashes leave. Get the picture?

So, what does this mean to Crystal? Well today we were at the hospital for over six hours. After meeting with her oncologist, they began to administer the Taxol slowly into her port. They wanted to go slower than usual to make sure she didn't have any allergic reactions. Thanks to a pre-dose of Atavan, steroids, and then Benadryl, she didn't have some of the side effects she was fearing: back pain and bouncing legs. She did have restless legs but not to the extent she was fearing.

Some of the effects this medicine has had on others are mouth sores, yellowing of the skin or eyes, unusual bleeding or bruising, being sensitive to sunlight, and high risk of infection. Not to mention the bouncing legs! After several hours at home tonight she is feeling better than expected. The oncologist told her the Benadryl would knock her out for about 24 hours. Well, she doesn't have bouncing legs...but she is bouncing off the walls. Must be the steroids. Lots of energy tonight!

She will not have to go back tomorrow for her white blood cell shot like she has with the first four treatments. This will give her only one trip to St. Vincent's a week for the next twelve weeks, unless she needs fluids. She has an open invitation to come and get a bag of juice at the hospital. This woman is not a big water drinker. I know the awful taste is constantly in her mouth...like taking a spoon of Vaseline. She has to be careful not to dehydrate. She is doing better, but not all-conference yet!

So, we enter the second phase. Big Red is in the rear view mirror... but so often nothing else can be seen in that mirror either. Although the room is full of cancer patients and caregivers....sometimes it just seems like no one is around. A room full of people...but no one there. I can't tell you how many times I have wanted to take her place...in the chair...in public...in the dark night...in the crowded room. Although Team Crystal is standing by her side there are times it seems it is only Crystal...nobody there.

Now before you quote one to me, let me quote one to you. *Joshua 1:5b says, "As I was with Moses, so I will be with you; I will never leave you nor forsake you."* My wife knows this to be true. This is the only way she has gotten this far...and the only way she gathers the strength to keep climbing in the chair. We know, as a family, that He will never forsake us. He will always be with us regardless of how quiet it may seem...just like he was with Moses (Knock, knock. Moses who?).

Our prayer for these next twelve weeks is that Crystal's body is not attacked as much by the Pacific Yew tree as the cancer cells, that she will have days and weeks where her energy level will be higher, where her throat will not be as sore, and the nausea will find somewhere else to go. We pray that each week when she goes to that crowded room at the hospital...she will always feel alone...with God! This fight has reminded us of what the true "pursuit of happiness" is all about.

Don't knock "my view from the front."

— **Bill**

Thirty-Five

When the Lights Go Out!

Sunday, November 1

Was Robert Redford on the field in a saggy uniform? Did a little guy run out and give someone a special wooden bat? Hollywood might not capture the moment but "when the lights go out" there has to be a story...a crazy finish to something that just got started. The family was there on another soggy Friday night...and we will talk about that night for years!

It was supposed to be Senior Night at BA, the last scheduled home game for Austin's team (playoff bound but finishing up the regular season). Why should we be surprised that the rains came again on Friday? Same song...next verse. Because of the driving rain, Senior Night would have to wait another week. Some mothers can't get their hair wet...so let's just play ball.

After about five minutes of action, our team had just scored it's second touchdown...up 13-0 on an out-manned opponent, preparing to kick the next point. Some of the fans had not even arrived to their seats, concession stand just getting rolling with the burgers and nachos, and the team with an expectation of another blow-out. Then it happened...the kick!

As the fourteenth point was rising into the damp night sky...as both teams started to make their way to the sideline...it happened! First a sizzle...then a loud boom! Sparks shot up in the air like the fourth of July. Matter of fact, Mr. P (who was at the game because he had a Thursday game that week) asked me, "Do they always have fireworks after every score?" Total and complete...darkness! No lights still on: not on the field, not on campus, not at the intersection in front of the school...darkness everywhere! What do you do "when the lights go out?"

You see our kicker...our 6' 4", 250 lb. kicker (with a college leg)... had kicked the ball into a transformer. The same transformer he hit earlier in the season during pre-game warm-ups that resulted in a delay of over an hour. A repeat performance...power has been knocked out! I mean nothing. No stadium lights. No public address system. No nachos. No exit signs. No street lights. Just sparks flying and children screaming. Halloween...a day early.

So, what do you do "when the lights go out?" Well, at BA you call the game. Send the visitors home. Playoffs start next week...let's go eat Mexican! The Gray's were watching the opening kick-off at 7:00...eating chips and salsa by 7:30! A story we will be telling for years.

Sometimes in a big football game, a heated battle between two physical opponents, someone on the field has their lights go out. It happens. When two strong forces collide something has to give... and sometimes it is "the lights." One minute you are there...the next, you are on the sidelines. What day is it? That feeling may last a few moments or a few weeks. One moment intense adrenalin...the next nothing but fog. How many fingers do I have up? On the field your legs are churning. Off the field you are standing on noodles. What is your name?

In life, so many people walk around as if living in a world of darkness...they can't see. Strength for the day is available...but they can't see. Peace, in troubled times, is there...but they can't see. Wisdom and direction, comfort and fellowship...but they can't find it. It is too dark! *John 12:46* says, *"I have come into the world as a light, so that no one who believes in ME should stay in darkness."*

It doesn't matter how physical your opponents are...He is the light. It doesn't matter how strong the force may seem against you... He is the light. The fog can't get too thick. The legs can't get too tired. The vision can't get too blurry. He is the light. And because He is the light, darkness disappears! His light shines everyday. Our eyes can stay fixed on Him. His name is Jesus! Those are things to remember!

Crystal will take her third round of Taxol on Tuesday. This chemo has been different on the body than the four doses of the "Red Stuff." The main difference is that the constant nausea feelings... are gone!! She has replaced that side effect with a constant flu like feeling, headaches and increasing soreness in her joints. Her left arm continues to hurt and we feel that is because of the nerves gradually coming back from the surgery. She still has a bad taste that will not go away, and for a few days after the treatments, she has no energy. Fatigue is her constant companion. So...she has to "turn out the lights" from time to time. There is indeed...rest for the weary.

This third quarter has been one of two physical opponents

attacking as hard as they can...and the body does suffer. Legs that were once strong...are not anymore. There are times when she feels stronger than others...and times when "strength" isn't even in the conversation. But as she will do on Tuesday...she keeps going back for more. We will be in single digits after the next visit. Progress is being made. It isn't time to turn out the lights just yet...still too much work to be done!

That, again, is "my view from the front"...as I turn out the lights.
– **Bill**

Thirty-Six

Not Today

Wednesday, November 11

Do you guys remember when you were in little league, back when the games were actually played during the summer months? That's a change. I can remember preparing all day for a game, getting the uniform on early in the day and making sure "everything" was just right. You know...getting my mind right. The world centered on those games...at least my world.

And do you remember the feeling when you saw the clouds starting to gather, and the rains starting to fall. At that age, I didn't know a more sinking feeling than to stand at the window, face to the glass, uniform just right...and hear the words, "Sorry, not today. Rain out!" You know what I am saying? Can you feel my pain? The world just didn't seem right when that happened...

As the games went from little league to college...the "not today" reasons became different. Not many rain outs on the gridiron but open dates were the norm. You know, the weeks when you had no game scheduled. Could mean a hard week of practice...or some rest for the legs depending on the time of season. Sometimes you welcomed the open date...so you could maybe get a win! It was a Saturday when everyone else seemed to be playing...but not you. Sorry, "not today."

We all experience those "not today" moments in our lives. Sometimes it is a cancelled flight...sometimes a phone call that doesn't come...or a trip to an empty mailbox. As I get older, those little league games have been replaced with...tee times. Rain and tee times don't go together very well...unless you are in Scotland or Ireland. Then, you play regardless of the weather.

Crystal went last week to St. Vincent's for her Tuesday treatment of Taxol. After hooking up her port (you know she has a port that is a 2009 model...very good mileage!), and checking her blood, the doctor said, "Not Today!" Because of her low white blood count she didn't get a treatment. A treatment would have put her in the hospital...already enough Taxol in the body. In layman's terms, she had received enough in two treatments to affect her body after three treatments. Therefore, not today.

As much as she dreads getting up on Tuesday mornings and being taken to "the chair"...to hear a "not today" (a rain out) was really not a bad thing. It would mean her body could get a week off. She could maybe not have as many days with headaches...a semi-normal week was ahead. Oh well, let's go eat lunch!

Yesterday, Crystal returned after an open date week. It was actually raining in Birmingham yesterday...a lot. Did I just see those dogs and cats lining up in pairs? Anyway, the port was activated...blood was pulled...tests were done. In came the doctor. "Well, Crystal, your numbers aren't much better. Sorry, Not Today." Two weeks in a row! "Sorry" and "not today" don't seem to go together. Who wouldn't want to be told they don't have to take the chemo?

I know in football you don't want your team to have back-to-back open dates. You lose your momentum. Your schedule that is so important...is thrown off. It defeats the purpose of the first open date. With chemo...it isn't that easy to decipher.

The oncologist assures us that the body is being attacked. She assures us that this is nothing to be alarmed about. Crystal's white blood count just hasn't gone up enough to show that her body can take another treatment. Nothing she has done to make it go down. Nothing she can do to make it go up. It is just her body reacting to the Taxol.

So...she waits...another week.

The good news about "not today" is that she is feeling better during the week. Friday night games are a scheduled event again. Food was actually prepared one night by her hands...a sight for sore eyes!! The good news about "not today" is that the doctor is finding out how her body handles the doses and is making adjustments. Next week we are supposed to be back on schedule. The plan at this moment is not to make up the treatments missed. Come on Doc...let's make sure that the cancer is still being attacked. Convince me!

A question for you: When was the last time you had a "not today" day? When was the last time you had a hope...only to see it dashed. When was the last time your bubble was burst? You know the verse I am thinking about today? It is found in **Hebrews 13:8, "Jesus Christ is the same yesterday and today and forever."**

You see, with Him, we never have to worry about a "not today" day. When you are looking out that window and it seems like the rain will never stop (uniform on but no game) just remember...He is the same in the rain and the sun! When you run into an "open date" in your life...when it seems everyone else is "playing" and you are not...He is the same and He hasn't changed! When you aren't sure why you can't keep the schedule you thought you were on...when God seems to change your plans in mid-stream...He is still the same! He is still in control...yesterday, today and forever.

Too many days I've been asked, "Are you writing tonight?", and the answer was "not today." Now you can see what I have seen over the last several days. A wife feeling semi-normal...that is a sight for sore eyes!

Today, this is "my view from the front."

– **Bill**

Thirty-Seven

A Roll and Cornbread

Sunday, November 15

She still hasn't gotten used to the "looks." Sometimes she is out with the bandanna...sometimes with the hat...and a few times you will find her with the wig. The wig with roots, but it is often too warm for the cranium! Yet...whatever the top dressing...she still gets the "looks."

She knows most people are just glad to see her. Others are surprised at her appearance. Yet there are some...who can't help but show an expression...of empathy. They know that whoever this lady is...bless her heart, she is going through a difficult time. Maybe they have been there themselves. Maybe they have seen a loved one in the same game. Maybe...just maybe...they wish they could help. The constant is always "the look." Not the same look we used to get when walking the mall with five young kids in tow (now that was a "different" look!).

She has also discovered that people will sometimes treat a bald-headed lady with kindness not expected. I am not talking about the cards....and meals...and tokens of love...that we continue to receive each week. I am talking about the other things that most of us don't see...but she sees.

It may be the man who goes out of his way to hold a door. It may be the lady who slows down enough to allow her to go in front at the checkout line. It could be the car in the next lane who allows her to move in front or the man at the shoe store who pulls a five-dollar coupon out of his pocket for her to use. All of them notice the head...and act with their heart.

It sometimes is the gentleman behind the counter at the end of the buffet. The choice of bread becomes no choice at all. He declares that for this customer...quietly of course...there will be no decision. She is going to get both breads...a roll and cornbread! Not asked for...but given anyway. A small act of grace...recognized by only one...but an act fresh from the heart! Sometimes you get more than you expect...even with cancer and a cap.

This week, Crystal felt good enough to travel to Austin's game in south Alabama. Two weeks removed from chemo will allow you to travel...but then you rest for two days. Yet the trade-off is sometimes worth it. She expects to be back in the chair this Tuesday to continue the game. Come on "white blood count." Rise up!

Anyway, after hearing that Mr. P's team won back home (Spain Park still rolling in the playoffs), we were able to witness more than we expected when we left home. Austin's team upset the number-one team in their league...and they are advancing to next week's championship game! He threw the game winner with under two minutes remaining and then intercepted their last-chance throw down the middle to seal the game. Crystal got to see it live...thanks to the white blood count. Sometimes you get more than you expect.

After taking a knee and letting the final seconds run out...Austin brushed aside the crowd celebrating on the field...and came over to me. Covered in mud...wet with sweat. I had a chance to hug a young man with tears in his eyes...and tears in mine. Crystal got a chance to see it live...through her tears. Sometimes you get more than you expect!

John 6:35 says, "Then Jesus declared, I am the bread of life. He who comes to me will never go hungry, and he who believes in me will never be thirsty." We have been reminded these past few days that we do indeed serve a God who is so gracious. He is the one to be praised for the success our boys have gotten to experience this fall. In Him...we truly never go hungry or thirsty. In Him...we always get more than we expect...or deserve! I thank Him this evening for the experience Crystal got to have last Friday night...even with cancer... even with the hat...and even with the low blood count.

Sometimes...you indeed get to have both "a roll and cornbread!"

Now you know "my view from the front."

– Bill

Thirty-Eight

Time to Self-Scout

Tuesday, November 24

In the game of football, and maybe in other sports as well, there always comes a time to look within...to see your team as the opponent sees you. To "self-scout." This is a time to evaluate what has happened over the last several games...to break it down play by play...to keep what has worked and to throw out what has not. It is a time where you stop...get away from the normal routine...and really take a look inside. Hopefully, you become a more efficient team with renewed focus...yet still striving for the goal. Sometimes it takes seeing things from the other side...to appreciate what you really have.

Over the last several days, I have had the opportunity to stop... and evaluate my team. With the season of Thanksgiving upon us, it is a good time for me to "self-scout"...and remind myself of what it looks like from the other side. Allow me to give you a glimpse of some thankful reminders I have been privileged to see.

Mr. P's season ended last week. He dressed for all (and played in a few) varsity games this fall....mostly without his parents in the stands. Chemo and Austin's senior season kept Crystal and I from attending all but a couple of his games...and there were many because of a great year that went deep into the playoffs. However, not once did son number two complain. He understood that sisters, sometimes sitting in the rain, had to replace mom and dad. I am thankful for his maturity...and love for his family...as well as their love for him.

Austin was in the locker room last week...minutes before his championship game...hooked up to an IV, getting much needed fluids. However, you would have had a hard time seeing him because he was surrounded by his teammates...in prayer. As a father, I could see the impact he has had on a new team...at a new school...making a positive difference. A decision last summer, bathed in prayer (much prayer) had turned into an experience our family will never forget. I am thankful for his boldness and courage...to initiate change...and to make a lasting difference at a new school his senior year.

Over the last several days I have gotten to see my children spend memorable moments with both sets of their grandparents. They may not realize...until later in life...how special those opportunities are in today's world. Age can bring wisdom...and wisdom is worth sharing....eliminating bumps down the road. I am thankful for the times when my children can spend time with the parents of their parents.

Crystal and her sister, with their mom in the kitchen...something that doesn't happen nearly as much as in years past...but it happened this week. Laughter shared...stories told (some stories for the umpteenth time)...and food prepared. The sight of our entire family in the kitchen...without enough seats...enjoying their time spent... and not looking to go to another room or TV. Those are things I am thankful for this week.

Brittany, Justin and their crazy Maltese Briley coming through the door and causing what was a calm, quiet evening to become chaos. I am thankful for them living minutes away. I am thankful for the visits...and the noise...and the maturity Brittany brings.

Bailey (the last eighth grader in Hoover to get a phone) looking at her first phone bill (that dad pays for) and seeing over 2000 text messages (and being proud)...is an experience for which I am thankful. A gift unexpected...but one definitely being used. She has grown up so much over the last few months.

Briana flipping a pie face down by accident on the kitchen floor...and causing laughter to break out....while mom is unaware in the other room...is a moment to be remembered. A moment for which to be thankful. Her being home this semester has been God ordained...even with the dirty clothes. All three of our girls have been a tremendous help to their mom. I am so proud to call each of them daughter...and so thankful for their giving spirit during this season.

The chair that Crystal crawled into again today....for the second week in a row... is something to be thankful for as well. Not so much the chair, but the reason for the chair...the healing that we trust is taking place in her body because of the medicine received while in the chair. I am thankful. She will be down for a couple of days but climbing back up as the week comes to an end...until she returns to the chair for the next treatment. I am thankful for healing.

Finally, the hardest one of all...so hard that it is literally difficult to type...cancer! Can one really be thankful for this awful disease? Can one be thankful for the pain and discomfort it causes? Can one be thankful that the body will forever be altered? Sometimes, I can honestly say...I don't know...and I am not even the one with the label.

However, I do believe in what **Psalm 95:2** says: *"Let us come before Him with thanksgiving and extol him with music and song."* I do know that because of cancer, we have seen God's hand at work in our lives. I do know that because of cancer, we have been blessed by so many that love my wife and our family. I do know that because of cancer, we have been able to see our children grow in dependence on Him. I do know that because of cancer, we have realized that we have so much to be thankful for.

We have experienced the music and song in our lives over these past few months like never before. For that I am thankful. We have an opportunity this week...any week...to take the time to "self-scout." To stop and look from the other side of the ball. We will continue to do that this week as we are reminded of the many blessings...of the many people...and of the many experiences...that we have to be thankful for this Thanksgiving.

I am blessed...and so thankful...to have "my view from the front."

– Bill

Thirty-Nine

Know and Be Still

Tuesday, December 1

I met a man today that I did not know. Have you ever been there? Have you ever felt the Lord "nudge" you in the direction of someone you didn't know...so that you could get to know them...if even for just a few minutes? That happened to me today. I met a quiet man with a story to tell. I took the first step...and was blessed in the end.

After breaking down the wall we so often put up...the wall of "I don't have time to visit"...he began to open up. A single father with three children. Two boys and one girl. A Baptist preacher from the country. Currently in a building program, where the members are cutting their own wood for the building. I told you it was country. A man with a story...

He began to talk about his oldest son, four years removed from high school...and a marine in Afghanistan. He told me of what his son was experiencing...while we hustle day to day in our own little world. His son is a medal-winning sharpshooter...and doing "recon" work in the mountains on the other side of the world. But one thing he said hit me like a ton of bricks. I had to let it sink in... and take effect. He said his son and one other marine recently did a "recon" mission, for thirty-one days...in the same spot...on the same mountain...never moving more than twenty feet...with temps in the teens!!

Now I would have a hard time staying still for thirty-one minutes. We live in an instant society. In football, we want to win...yesterday. In banking, results come when relationships are built...but we get impatient. We all have microwave ovens...a drive-thru on every corner...and Eggo waffles for breakfast in the toaster. We live too fast. Can you imagine being still for "thirty-one days?" That marine was still...so that we can know our busy world is protected.

That marine was still...and knew what was expected of him. That marine was still...and knew his strength would come from prayers being lifted up by a single dad...in the country. Crystal was still today...in the chair.

Crystal was still today...and knew the medicine had to go into the veins...for healing to have a chance. Crystal was still today...for several hours...knowing when she got up she would have her chemo visits down to five!! It is tough to sometimes wait...

Crystal has spent a little bit longer in the mirror lately...being still. She has noticed that her face isn't framed by eyebrows...like it used to be. She knows...that this is another side effect of the chemo. So she sits...and for a while she looks...but knows they will return.

Is it as hard for you, as it is for us? To just sometimes sit...and know? I don't mean for thirty-one days...or even for thirty-one minutes...unless you feel led by the "nudge" of the Lord. Are you ever reminded by the scripture verse...you know the one. **Psalm 46:10... "Be still and know that I am God..."**

Today I was reminded to just be still...and know. Reminded because of the visit to the chair by my eyebrow-less wife. (Baby, you are down to one hand...count 'em. FIVE!) I was reminded today because of the sweet friend that sat still in the waiting room...with a book in her hand and love in her heart...for my wife. I was reminded today because of the man I did not know...and the story of the son... being still.

I challenge you to take some time tomorrow to "be still and know" regardless of your circumstances...or the clock on the wall. Because of cancer...and because of our many friends who care...we have been reminded to be still. To know...that He is indeed God!

Still..."my view from the front!"

– **Bill**

Forty

Eye Black and Stick 'um

Sunday, December 6

Regardless of which direction we look, colors bring messages. Each one is tied to a thought that reminds us of something – some from times gone by and others from today...or yesterday. My son goes to a "blue" ribbon school. We drive through "yellow" caution lights everyday. The media will tell you it is time to go "green." At church this morning, I shook hands with a lady who had the same color bracelet on her arm that I have on mine...a "pink" cancer bracelet (her mother is battling the same opponent as Crystal).

Yesterday we watched a young man play quarterback from Florida with a message on his cheeks...a scripture verse written on eye "black." Eye Black, originally designed to keep the glare of the sun out of a players eyes when playing a day game, has been transformed into an easy way to project your message to millions of people...or to just one. Tim Tebow has used his cheeks to remind the football world of the promises from God's word. In the SEC championship game, his verse was from *John 16:33* which reminded us that we *"will have trouble,"* but to take heart because He has overcome the world!

Tebow has used multiple verses over his career, such as **Philippians 4:13** and the promise that *"I can do everything through Him who gives me strength."* Those "eye blacks" have spoken to so many over the years. Personally, it would have been good if he had used at some point **Ephesians 6:1**, *"Children obey your parents,"* or **Proverbs 22:6**, *"Train up a child in the way he should go."* Those two verses would have spoken to the children...and to the children raising children... but that is another story for another time.

Eye black has come a long way since I was a player. We didn't have the peel-off kind that you put on like a postage stamp. We had a tube of black grease that reminded you of something from a body shop. I also played during a time when coaches would have thought you were showboating to put it on your face. But as my college career began, there was another player who had everyone's attention...well, at least mine, and many others....on the television. He used enough eye black...and stick 'um...to grease several cars. His name was Fred Biletnikoff.

Biletnikoff played in the sixties and seventies and was a Super Bowl MVP and Hall of Fame receiver. As a result of his storied career, the award for the best receiver in college football today is called the Biletnikoff Award. As a receiver growing up...he was my Tim Tebow. He would have stuff under his eyes and stuff on his socks. He would rub his socks before every play and have enough artificial substance on his hands...that when the ball came his way...the catch was always made. Freddy 'B'...my hero! No scripture verses, but someone I could relate to...slow and small...but a clutch performer when his number was called.

Let me tell you why this is important to me tonight. Several reasons come to mind. First of all, my hero today is not very big...

and she is not very fast...but she is a clutch performer! She can't go deep and get behind the coverage...but on third down she is going to get open for the first! She also has made an impact on a lot of people...some she has not even met (I have never met Fred either).

Second, she is wearing socks a lot these days...especially of late. She doesn't have stick 'um on them...but since she hasn't felt good enough to get out much...she "sticks" around the house. The Taxol this week has caused her to have some head aches and some stomach battles. After a Thursday trip to see Austin's final high school game... she has been regulated to the bench (couch and bed) all weekend. She made the play on Thursday...although she should have been on the sidelines.

Finally, I have not seen her in eye black, but she is resting in the promise that Tebow advertised on Saturday. Because of the promise that Jesus said we "would" have trouble (not "may" have or "could" have), she believes. He said we "will." Because of this she also believes the rest of the verse. She has *"taken heart,"* and she knows also that *"He has overcome the world."* Those are words anyone can rest in tonight.

Freddy "B" had a major influence on me when I was young. Tim Tebow has had a major impact on my boys in their young years. Like Tebow...Crystal can and will get through this tough time...because her eyes, like his above the black, are looking up!

Without the glare from the sun, that is "my view from the front."
– Bill

Forty-One

It's the Little Things...

Saturday, December 19
(another entry...long overdue)

We often find ourselves repeating our replies: "She is doing fine" or "Hanging in there" or "Still fighting." All are true...but more of a big picture response. Some are looking for more details, while others just want you to know they care. One thing is for sure, we have gotten used to the constant inquiries...and are blessed to have so many concerned.

However, there are other signs that often go unnoticed...except by our family. Some are better left to the walls of our home. Others... let me say...are worth sharing. Anyone who has had a loved one go through this series of treatments can probably relate. Let me share some of the "little things" we have noticed.

They say the patient will get what is called "chemo brain." Not sure if that has been accurately defined in a book but our family has seen (and heard) what appears to be the result. You hear a lot of the same questions repeated. On Tuesdays, after she leaves the hospital, whoever drives "Ms. Daisy" home will have to repeat themselves several times. It doesn't matter how "s-l-o-w'" you speak...or how direct...get ready to repeat! It gets better as the week goes by but "chemo brain" is alive and well...and sometimes will bring a smile to your face! Little things.

Another sign is the shrinking of the body. Her arms and legs are where one would notice the most change. The chemo attacks and tears down. The appetite seldom shows up. The fatigue is constant. Therefore, the weight begins to drop and the "guns" and "hams" become smaller...the clothes a little looser. Little things.

Sometimes you notice that the ability to carry out physical tasks becomes a little more of a challenge. Attacking stairs...either up or down...is a little more careful. Picking up things takes a little more concentration. Just this week, Crystal was taking a pie from the hands of our neighbor (in our kitchen) who had brought us dinner... and pulled a Briana!! Yep, the pie did a one and a half onto the floor! Clean up on aisle four! So much for dessert. I don't know whose face was more shocking...Crystal's or our neighbor's. Chocolate pies don't ever seem to make it to our table. Little things.

Earlier this week, Mr. P was the recipient of a little thing. He was being taken to school by his mother (out of necessity). First time in a while she had driven in the early morning. Let me just say two words...white knuckles! Mr. P said he had never seen his mom drive the van like that! She wasn't Danica Patrick...but she wasn't far off. As you can imagine, he was very glad to get to school...in one piece. Thank goodness that was a little thing.

One little thing that means so much is that Crystal is now down to three treatments of chemo! Can I get an AMEN somebody?! Since the last entry, she has had two more treatments. Her numbers are up enough to continue but not where they should be. We are seeing the cumulative effects of Taxol...but only for three more trips. Then she will get her game plan for the fourth quarter...radiation. Amen for little things.

Finally, during this season of the year, you can't help but look for the "little things" that mean so much. Often the things that are little have the greatest impact on our lives. Of course, the "little" baby in the manger takes center stage to so many. It should go without saying that our Christmas season is more special this year!

Let me give you one other "little" to think about. Remember the following verse the next time you go out your front door early in the morning to get the paper. If you are like me, you will probably walk on some damp, brown, cold, stiff grass to retrieve the daily fish wrapper. Think of this: in **Matthew 6:30** we find, *"If that is how God clothes the grass of the field, which is here today and tomorrow is thrown into the fire, will he not much more clothe you, O you of little faith?"...*

Because of all the "little things" we have learned and experienced during this journey, our family's faith has grown. You can't hear the words we have heard...see the things we have seen...and feel the love we have felt...without your faith growing! I pray your faith grows because of the "little things" in your life.

That's again "my view from the front"...and it is not a "little thing."
– Bill

Forty-Two

Upon Further Review...

Friday, December 25

In football, those three words can make an entire stadium and viewing audience...come to a halt. The official will either state that the previous play stands as is or the prior result will be reversed. Either way, one side of the field will be disappointed for the second time...or be given "new life" with a reversal. On the other side, that team will hope for a confirmation of what they have just celebrated...or will have their smiles ripped from their faces by a man in a booth. It brings the game to a halt, but has the intention of making every thing right.

As this Christmas Day comes to an end, I can't help but pause...and give the past twenty-four hours "a further review." To say this was a special Christmas for our family would be an understatement. Because of Crystal's treatments and her "after effects," our family opted not to travel to visit other family members out of state but instead celebrated at home with just our five children and one son-in-love. It was a bittersweet decision...but one that our family will remember for a long time.

The day started like most of America with Crystal and I in the kitchen cooking more food than our crew could eat (we were blessed to receive some assistance from some special friends!). Except for fighting a headache most of the day, Crystal made sure that her children had a day to remember. Brittany purchased a new camera for her and Justin, so we hope to have some new photos to place in our album. There is nothing like the smell of a kitchen on Christmas morning...with the warm sounds of a crackling fireplace...mixed in, with one last day of Christmas music in the background.

Before the gifts could be unwrapped, Bailey read "The Story" from Luke 2 – one final opportunity to stop and have a "further review." As we discussed the events of that first Christmas evening, Brittany reminded our family of Matthew's version. This was also the focus of the service we attended last night. It was a special way to prepare for this day!

Before we went to a Christmas Eve service, we met a special family for an early dinner. One of their four children, Caleb, is a six year old with a heart of gold. As our two families surrounded a long table of Mexican food, I asked Caleb what he wanted for Christmas...an answer he had already made clear to his parents weeks earlier. He said, "A Build-a-Bear gift certificate and a small pink bracelet that would fit him with Ms. Crystal's name on it...so he could 'pway' for her!" I don't have to tell you how many eyes were watering after that statement. We could have had church right there over a fajita (upon further review...)!

We then went to the service. The church we attended has about a three hundred yard walk from the parking lot to the doors of the worship center. It was extremely windy last night. So picture Crystal trying to get inside without "losing her wig." I mean we had her surrounded...like secret service agents. Some children were in front to "block." Others were in back to "scoop and score" if necessary. Crystal was looking down to try and stay under the wind. I had my hand on her neck...and hair...the entire way. It may have flipped over but it wasn't going to fly off !!

All the while we were trying to get her inside in one piece, we were constantly being told by ushers "Welcome" and "Merry Christmas." If they had only known what was on our minds...and her head! After a visit to the ladies room to "straighten and secure," we had a wonderful worship experience.

One final review if you will...

As mentioned earlier, the message from last night was focused on **Matthew 1:23, "The virgin will be with child and will give birth to a son, and they will call Him Immanuel" - which means, "God with us."**

Christmas is a time of year when our focus is on children...and the wonder in their eyes...and sometimes out of their mouths! It is also a time for us to focus on "the Child" that came to be with us! Just like in the review of a football play, Immanuel came to bring us "new life" that can never be reversed! He came to give a reason to "celebrate" a hope in Him! He should bring us to a "halt" on more days than just this one! He doesn't sit in a booth...but He does sit on a throne!

As this day comes to a close, and another Christmas is in the book, the experiences our family has witnessed was worthy of me taking another look...a "further review."

The play stands...and that is "my view from the front!!"

– Bill

Forty-Three

Different...But the Same.

Wednesday, December 30

Team Crystal, we are down to our final treatment! The third quarter of this battle is finally coming to a close. After yesterday's trip to "the chair," Crystal will go back next Tuesday for her last scheduled chemo treatment! (That felt good to type – the word "last" and "chemo" go well together.) Her numbers again were up enough and they gave her the green light. One more time to put the poison in her port. A great way to bring in the New Year!

She will then have a week or so off before starting the fourth quarter...daily radiation for five to six weeks. We understand the side effects will be nothing compared to the chemo...except for some tender skin, discoloration, and more fatigue. The persistent headaches, compliments of some medicine mixed in the drip to keep her from being nauseous, will hopefully disappear. Suffice it to say.... things will look and feel a little different.

Different...that word has continued to surface this week in many ways. The week started Sunday with a visit from my brother and his family, along with my parents. They all drove over from Georgia to spread Christmas cheer. Richard's kids...my kids. A room full of Gray's. All the same...but different...in a good way.

When you are inside "the circle", or around when Crystal is feeling "giddy," you get the privilege of seeing Crystal's new look on top. Her hair is coming back in...slowly...but still different. She has a fine, low look to her scalp. It is coming back with a mixture of white (or grey, if we are honest) and black. I would call it "houndstooth." My fellow bankers in Tuscaloosa would like that terminology. After all these years of the same on top...she is now different.

I sat last night at a basketball game and listened as a neighbor talked about the differences in her children. As my children get older, the differences begin to show as well. All from the same parents... but all very different. I will give you an example from an incident after last night's game. I took the boys by a unique hamburger joint and called to see if Briana or Bailey needed a take-out. Crystal was asleep on the couch. And just like clockwork, around midnight...she came to life. (Her usual Tuesday routine after a treatment.)

Anyway, here is what I heard from my daughter on the phone: "Yes, bring me the veggie burger. Grilled portabello mushroom and eggplant, with Swiss cheese, caramelized vidalia onions and roasted red peppers on a toasted onion Kaiser roll...and add feta cheese." Do what?!! Now that may not mean much to you today, but it proved to me that each of my children are indeed different. I have heard of marching to the beat of a different drum...but that is an entire band!

Now before any vegetarians take up their pens, let me say, it isn't the fact of the veggie burger being veggie. It is the fact of the veggie burger being ordered! She didn't get that from her mom or dad (where's the Beef?!). So much alike...but so different. Each of them hearing their own music, which is not a bad thing at all, as long as there is still a connection with what is ultimately important in life.

The scriptures even speak of how each of us are different and yet the same. *I Corinthians 12:4-5 says, "There are different kinds of gifts, but the same spirit. There are different kinds of service, but the same Lord."* Aren't you glad there is not another you? Aren't you glad God made all of us different...but the same? Kinda like Baskin-Robbins – so many choices. Different....but the same. Some of us are arms, some are legs, some are eyes, and some are toes. But together we are a Body!

Life can sometimes become monotonous. We can get caught in the same routine every day. We can find ourselves just going through the motions...with no meaning...with no benefit. Getting plugged in every Tuesday...to wait on the next Tuesday.

Crystal's fourth quarter will be different. Looking above her eyes...I see something different. Our children have each handled this experience differently and will see life a little differently as well. I am not ready to put a mushroom inside some bread just yet. However, I am glad my kids have reminded me that God made us all different... yet the same!

It's different...but it is still "my view from the front."

– Bill

Forty-Four

An Empty Chair and Icing in the Carpet

Wednesday, January 6

Yesterday I took Crystal to St. Vincent's for her final round of chemo. She went through the same entrance, walked the same hallway, sat in the same waiting room, moved to the same exam area, and got stuck the same way with her port...just like she has done for twenty weeks. That is five months...if you have been counting. The same faces...nurses and doctors...greeted her. Only, this time it was different.

We met with her oncologist and again I asked some pointed questions. As we get closer to the end of this game...I can't help but think about the next one. How do we know all this has done any good? What will she do next? Will it resurface...somewhere else? Is there not any "final exam" to be taken? Again, we got the same answers as last time. Only, this time it was different.

The nurses, bless their hearts, were again in a positive frame of mind. The nurses that work in the cancer area....are special people. They knew that this was the last time for Crystal to have the poison pumped in her veins. They were encouraging. They were funny. They were excited...to be able to assist in the healing process. Only, this time it was different.

After getting her blood work done, with her numbers up closer to normal, they moved Crystal to her chair. As usual, the room was full of cancer patients...fighters! Some looked familiar. Some smiled. Some were new faces. Some with no expression at all. Some of the patients were alone...and some had support. Some were just beginning their ballgame...their fight. The room was the same as always. Only, this time it was different.

When you get to the final treatment, it is customary for there to be a celebration. It doesn't have to be elaborate...but somebody is going to party! We discovered that you can make these nurses party by bringing an Edgar's strawberry cake! They attacked that thing like they hadn't eaten in weeks. It looked like a bomb had gone off in that box. Etiquette is not a factor when it comes to an unattended cake sitting on an exam table. About the only way to know something had been eaten...was the icing in the carpet! The "pink strawberry" tint in the room...made everything a little different.

I have taken more pictures in my life than I can recall. At 5:15 this past Tuesday, I took a picture that I will remember for the rest of my life. As pics go, it is very pale in color. It's subject sits on a hard floor inside a partitioned off room. The surface is made of vinyl and has a place to raise your legs. Some in the room were still occupied but this one was empty. The empty chair!! I might need to get an 8 x 10 of that one. That empty chair made everything different.

Daniel 4:2 says, "It is my pleasure to tell you about the miraculous signs and wonders that the Most High God has performed for me." As we left the hospital on Tuesday, I couldn't help but think of all the things that will forever be ingrained in our minds about this battle. Many you have read about in these pages. Some you will never know. Two that will always have a special place in my heart...will be an empty chair and icing in the carpet. Signs that will give me an opportunity to tell people about the wonders of our Most High God!

Those are signs you can only see...with "my view from the front."
– Bill

Forty-Five

Four Fingers

Thursday, January 28

On nearly every sideline, in nearly every stadium, you will see it. It always happens at the end of the third quarter...and the beginning of the fourth! The players will raise their hands with the "Four Fingers" pointed high. The crowd of supporters will raise their fingers as well. In some places coaches will also raise the "Four Fingers" high! It signifies that we have ONE final quarter to play and that we will give our best...finish strong! The fourth quarter belongs to the strong. We have paid the price....we are strong...finish strong!

I realize (because I have been reminded constantly) that it has been three weeks since my last entry. I could give you many reasons. Some of them merit your patience...some of them don't. However, I will tell you what has been on our minds since the last entry. Just like the players on the sideline...we are beginning the fourth quarter. So, I will give you the "four" fingers of our constant thoughts over the last few weeks...as we enter the fourth.

First, over the past couple of weeks Crystal has been dealing with a constant pain in her left side. We have been to the hospital on three different occasions to address the issue. Once was in the emergency room...til about 1:00 am (Can we get someone to look into the staffing of our emergency rooms? It is called an "emergency room" for a reason...hello?) Anyway, we have been blessed that every scan or x-ray has come back negative. Good news! Still, the pain persists. So, we press on to find the source...with the help of a pill or two from time to time. Finish Strong!

Second, Crystal met today with the Radiology Oncologist. We now have a game plan for the fourth quarter. She will have twenty-eight sessions of radiation. She will go daily, Monday through Friday, for just over five weeks. She is to start next week. The sessions will last about twenty minutes. She has been told the side effects are nothing compared to the chemo. More fatigue...and a sensitive left upper chest area...but better than chemo! Finish Strong!

Third, Crystal has always been a lady of small stature. Only now, that stature is getting smaller by the hospital visit. She continues to lose weight...down fifteen pounds since opening kick-off. There are several factors in the "loose Levis." Not feeling well...leads to a mind that sometimes wonders...which leads to a loss of appetite...which compounds the previous loss of taste buds from the chemo...which results in a smaller shadow on the wall. She has always talked about losing weight but I don't think this is the route you really want to go. So, as a result...I have gained what she has lost! (That is another story.) Finish strong!

Fourth, are the broken legs. We were sitting in the waiting area the other day at the hospital and a couple of patients walked by with broken legs. The comment was made, "wouldn't it be nice...to only have a broken leg?"

This journey has taught us to appreciate the little things...to not take things for granted quite so much. We all have this problem. The world at times looks so dim...so tough. But it is all relative. The same time we think about wanting a broken leg, their is someone else looking at us wishing they were able to make it to the fourth quarter. Their results, their tests, their consultations...were far worse than what we have heard and seen. Oh, to just have...someone else's battle. Finish Strong!

Those are some of the thoughts that have been on our minds for the past few weeks. However, make no mistake. Our God is faithful! He is in control! We don't always understand...but we trust. We read scripture...and we trust Him.

One scripture that reminds us of our thoughts is found in *Deuteronomy 11:18. It says, "Fix these words of mine in your hearts and MINDS; tie them as symbols on your hands and bind them on your foreheads."* In other words, listen to what is written in scripture... and remember it! Listen to what the Lord speaks to you...and keep it front and center! Place them in your heart...and your minds!

The fourth quarter has begun. Team Crystal...get your fingers up! This quarter is ours! We will finish STRONG!!

As you already know...that's "my view from the front!"
– Bill

Forty-Six

Whoever has the Pen Last Wins

Monday, February 1

This coming Wednesday, the fourth quarter will start for Team Crystal. She will go daily to St. Vincent's for twenty-eight treatments of radiation. Better than twenty-nine!! After the day she had today, I couldn't help but think of board rooms in banks and staff rooms in field houses. In everyone of those rooms, you will find the same tools: dry erase boards and grease pens. Whoever has the pen last... wins!

It is common to hear margins and rates being discussed in the financial field. The pen can show the rise of one and the fall of the other. Some things are out of a banker's control. Some things make him grit his teeth...and hang on. However, the wise banker plans ahead with conservative thinking. His pen shows promise down the road. He holds tight to the pen in tough times...so that in the end... he has an opportunity to win!

I have never met a football coach who didn't have an answer. Put one on the board...and he will draw one up. Whether it is going up the board or down the board, he can always make one seem to work against any defense. He can also have one too many to block...if given the chance. Any one worth his salt will always have an answer. Every coach knows...he who has the pen last wins!

Personally, I think too much of the coaching profession has relied solely on the power of the pen...and not the person. I know coaches who coach young men...grow young men...and mentor young men through the game of football. They are in the profession not because of the pen...but because of the heart. Those are the ones I want spending time with my boys. Grow young men with your pen and your witness. Don't just draw plays. You CAN have it both ways. (Now I will get off my soapbox.)

So Crystal went this morning and found out what angle the radiation would have to attack her body. After marking her body up with "the pen" like a third and long play, she got some bad news. There would have to be some adjustments made in the front in order for the radiation to reach it's desired locations. So, a trip to the plastic surgeon was then taken. Now she has driven down highway 280 hundreds of times...but never to be "deflated!" She went in perfectly balanced...and came out leaning to the left! Lean with it... rock with it!!

Then came another trip back to St. Vincent's to get some more body art. She went from a pass play to looking like a road map. I now have my very own "living" GPS system...that leans a little left! What a day!! The doctors now have a pattern drawn where they will concentrate the radiation and it will only have an effect on the parts that need to be attacked. The things that ladies have to go through... ladies who are breast cancer survivors...in order to again look and feel like a lady. Can I say this? Those ladies...my wife...are tough!!

The doctors marked with the pen...in order for Crystal to have an opportunity to win. This is the last quarter, and the pen has come out...so that in the end she can finish strong! Whoever has the pen last...wins!

Revelation 21:5 says, "He who is seated on the throne said, 'I am making everything new' Then he said, 'Write this down, for these words are trustworthy and true.'" We woke up this morning with the promise that our God makes everything new! You can write that down. It is trustworthy...and true! He is seated on the throne, in control. No matter what your circumstances are...no matter how much you may not understand...regardless of the rates, or the defense in front of you...He is in control! He has asked us to write it down!

With the help of the doctors...and the direction of divine intervention...soon Crystal will be leveled out and balanced again. Soon she will be finished with the twenty-eight. Soon she will be "like new." She is the one with the pen...on her chest. She is the one who will win!

Sleeping next to my GPS...and trying to figure out..."my view from the front!

– **Bill**

Forty-Seven

A Chance to Win in the Fourth

Saturday, February 13

Years ago I worked for a coach (a "mountain of a man" coach) with a tender heart. He knew his football...still does...and he always wanted to put his team in a position. Some would say he was conservative...didn't take enough chances. Some would say his offenses were boring...didn't attack as often as they should. But... he had a plan. He always had a plan. He would tell his team... repeatedly just to hold on. All we want, guys, is "a chance to win in the fourth! Play to give yourselves a chance...a chance to win in the fourth!" The man had wisdom...and he won more than he lost.

Crystal is playing the fourth quarter as I type. She has finished the eighth treatment of radiation...with twenty more to go. She is playing to put her self in position...to have "a chance to win in the fourth!" We don't understand everything her doctor is doing, everything she is planning, but we trust she has wisdom. I know her doctor is being lifted up in prayer...for God to give her wisdom...so Crystal will have "a chance to win in the fourth!"

Last week I went into the room where the radiation takes place. For those who haven't ever been inside, I will try to describe. After entering through a door that reminded me of the door on our vault at the bank, I turned the corner to see a massive machine. This machine, which looked like it weighed a ton, was in the center of the room. It hung out over a table where the patient would lay down.

Each patient, Crystal included, lays inside of a form fitting just for them. This fitting is like a cast...or a cocoon...or a cradle. It keeps the part of the body that is being radiated (is that a word?) from moving. Each one is formed just for that one single patient. They hang all around the walls. You come in...they grab your cradle...you lay down, and they go to work.

Of course, like every other step in this journey, you lay mostly uncovered, exposed to the world...or at least the lab technicians. (Crystal lost her modesty a long time ago in this game.) One unique thing about this place is the ceiling. On the ceiling is a beautiful picture...a 3-D picture of some tropical vacation paradise. I have never been to a tanning bed, so I don't know if this is common or not. But I do know...this is one expensive tan that Crystal gets everyday. Although she will not have the bronze beach body you would expect with this picture...she will have the "first day on the beach" burn!

The radiation treatments last about fifteen to twenty minutes each day. The Bruno Cancer Center has this thing down to a science. Crystal has a scheduled time each day that is assigned to her. She valet parks at the door, gets greeted by the friendliest valets in the city who always call her by name, and goes to her changing room. She waits to be called back. Those waits can be quick...or can last a while...but they are always in God's perfect timing.

The other ladies she has met in the waiting room have made her feel blessed at times...and at times have made her feel worse. Everyone has their own story and all are looking to the future... with anticipation, and for an ear to listen. These sessions with other patients bring home the reality of what she is going through. Some... no, all...are just wanting "a chance to win in the fourth!"

Crystal will begin to feel more and more tender in her left chest area and back. She has to put this lotion, special lotion, on her front and back three times a day. The back because the radiation machine moves all the way around her body. The left side of her throat is beginning to get sore because it too is in the area being treated. She will go from rare...to medium-well...to very well done by the time this is all over. Her skin will get hard and tough...like your grandparent's luggage...and then months later will come back to a more normal texture.

Her left side is still bothering her. She has a constant pain just below her ribs. It doesn't get better standing up or sitting down. It is the same in the morning or late at night. We are probably looking at doing a PET scan in the next week...just to try one more time to get some answers. Even though every answer so far has been positive... the pain is still there.

In reality, our pain is nothing compared to the pain our Savior went through on this earth. *John 13:7* has Jesus replying, *"You do not realize now what I am doing, but later you will understand."* He just wanted His followers to keep working until the fourth quarter. They would understand in time. Their understanding would make sense in the end. If only they would take to heart what He was telling them... and trust Him...in time they would be victorious! All of these trips to the Cancer Center are for one reason.

All of these steps are for one goal. All of these scans...and tests...and lotions...and tropical pictures...are for one purpose. All Team Crystal wants is to have "a chance to win in the fourth!" And Win we will!

Even though it is "pinker"...it is still "my view from the front!"

– Bill

Forty-Eight

Under the Hat... into the Cup

Wednesday, February 24

Like a ton of bricks, a slap in the face, or a bucket of cold water. Frozen in time...catch my breath. What did she say? All of those could describe Crystal's feelings today at Publix. Maybe now I know why she doesn't like to go to the store. I'll set it up...

As Crystal was checking out with a few groceries, the young cashier asked her, "Ma'am, would you like your senior discount?". Say what?! Crystal was sandwiched in between two older ladies, one that just checked out and one that was beginning to put her items on the sliding belt. All she could say was, "Well, how old do I have to be for the "senior discount?" Again, be careful what you ask for. The girl by the register said, "Sixty."

Now Crystal wasn't aware that Wednesday's at Publix are "Senior Discount Days." Nor was she aware that in her "little blue hat" she looked sixty! You can imagine what question I got when I got home today. "Do I look sixty?"...excuse me?!

One quick PSA. Don't imply to a woman that just went through chemo and is currently going through radiation that she looks older. Doesn't make for a fun time at the house. Now, there is nothing wrong with anyone looking sixty...unless that person is forty-eight.

Crystal has been fond of her light blue lid since losing her covering. She bounces back and forth from the wig...to the lid. However, she has a friend that has been pushing her to go natural...to let 'em see what is under the hat." Now, just maybe, she will start to consider that option a little more strongly. The "Jamie Lee Curtis Look" may be better than getting asked about discounts...I'm just saying.

As the fourth quarter moves on, she has completed sixteen treatments of radiation. Along with the mounting fatigue, guys, it is like checking your steaks on the grill. Each time you raise the lid... or pull back her shirt...you see a little change in the color and texture. Only problem is she can't turn over to the other side with a set of tongs. She still looks at the tropical paradise on the ceiling in that room...and pushes toward number twenty-eight.

The pain in her left side is still a constant. Today, she visited a urologist about a test result that came back last Friday...one with some red blood cells that were found in what went "into the cup." The doctors are still baffled by what could be causing the pain...but they are still searching for answers. We will get the results from today's tests back in a couple of days. We don't expect it to be any different than all the others...clear with no sign of cancer!

In order to get a little better sleep at night, she has gone to "the Patch." A four by four adhesive with a cool gel that she puts on her side at night. Twelve hours on and twelve hours off. No nicotine in this baby, but just something to take the edge off "the thorn in her side" until we get answers (or as Jerry Clower would say, "some relief!").

You know, on any football team trying to win in the fourth many will probably be playing with pain. They will probably start to get weary of doing the same things over and over...play after play. However, in order to be successful, in order to finish off the opponent...it is vital to stick to the plan. And it is that group of teammates, that cohesive group, which will sustain each other. They gather strength from each other. That is what makes a team so special!

Let me try and tie this all together with a verse from "The Plan" for our life. In *Isaiah 46:4* it reads, *"Even to your old age and gray hairs I am He, I am He who will sustain you. I have made you and I will carry you. I will sustain you and I will rescue you."* Did you hear that? Let it sink in.

Young or old...He is He. Young or old...He will sustain you. He will never get tired. He doesn't need to look at a medical test. He made you in order to carry you. He has to Hold YOU. He will not only sustain you in the fourth quarter...he will rescue you! Anyone who is rescued...Wins!!

Games are decided in the fourth quarter. Twelve treatments remain. So, before the last whistle sounds I am sure Crystal will still make people wonder what is "under the hat"...and I am sure she will be asked to put something else "into the cup." Not to worry though...He will sustain her!

Looking for more discounts...and looking at "my view from the front."

– Bill

Forty-Nine

I Saw it on Her Face

Thursday, March 4

Proverbs 27:19 says, "As water reflects a face, so a man's heart reflects a man."

We see them everyday. It starts from the moment we get out of bed. When we pass them going down the stairs for breakfast. When we pull onto a busy street. When we walk into a classroom. When we go to work...or to shop...or to play. Sometimes we see our own... sometimes we see others. But we still see them...daily.

Faces...other's faces...our faces.

Late in the fourth quarter of a football game, I want to see faces. I want to see faces of confidence. I want to see teammates gathered together...finding a way...showing confidence in their faces. It helps when those who support are also showing confidence. It is an expression that feeds off itself ! Show me confidence...I will probably show you confidence in return. We can get this done! We can win it in the fourth! The faces of confidence!

Crystal is six treatments from being finished with her radiation.

(Did you hear the angels rejoicing as you read that last sentence?) After tomorrow...her twenty-third trip in this quarter...she will have one week left. It is late in the fourth and we are looking for confident faces! Show me confidence. Show her confidence. Don't get in the huddle...unless we can see your confident face.

This week, I was reminded of other faces that we see.

There are some faces of confusion. I have seen them, in places I didn't expect them to be. Some are confused about their purpose. Some are confused about a result...that wasn't like they had planned. Some are confused about the future...it shows in their faces. It shows in their attitudes. It shows in their relationships. (On the side of Crystal's giant radiation machine is a reminder about how God is not a God of confusion. She reads it everyday.) Don't get in the huddle... with a confused face.

There are faces of contentment. Crystal and I had dinner with a sweet couple who both had faces of contentment. Their life was a reflection of contentment in their God, in His plan. Although they have never experienced cancer, they traveled a road just as bumpy as ours. They played a game just as hard as this one. However, their faces were content. They had a peace...in an unpredictable world. Something that comes from a life of "God Explained" experiences. They can get in our huddle...with faces of contentment.

There are also faces of concern. Crystal sees them everyday in a crowded waiting room. She says one of the things that is so hard about this fourth quarter has been the daily walk through this room. It hurts. The patients hurt. Their families hurt. Cancer hurts.

The large salt water fish tank in the middle may make it calm but it doesn't hide the fear. She tries to smile at some who make eye contact, but too many times there is no smile in return. Just faces...

of concern.

A lady today caught her eye. They were both in a smaller waiting area next to a changing room. Crystal told me she could tell it was her first time to get treatment. Crystal said, "I saw it in her face!" She had a face of concern, of fear. Her face was close to tears. Crystal knew it was the first time because she had the same look twenty- two treatments ago.

It is easier for a team to win in the fourth when that team has been there before. Crystal will be able to get in any huddle at the hospital after this game and look those players in the eye...with confidence. That verse in Proverbs tells me that our faces reflect what is in our hearts. You can't hide it in your face that God is in control...so reflect it!

Look confusion in the face with a heart of confidence! Look contentment in the face...knowing God is so good...with a heart of confidence! Look concern in the face with a promise that God is in control...and with a heart of confidence! That's the type of faces I want in my huddle in the fourth.

See it in His face…in His huddle!

Huddle Up...and see "my view from the front."
– **Bill**

Fifty

A Drive to Remember

Tuesday, March 9

Every coach has one. Some are written on small paper. Some are written on large cardboard. Some are hand-written. Some are typed. Some smear when it rains. Some are laminated. Some have multiple colors...key words...front and back. Some are written in their minds from experience. But every coach has one.

They are used during the entire game. Actually, they are formulated during the week leading up to the game. They are important during every quarter, but mostly late in the fourth. They are...Game Plans.

Every situation is covered. Run. Pass. Screens. Draws. Misdirection. First and ten calls. Regular downs. Second and long. Third and long. Third and short. Short yardage. Goal line calls. Gadget plays. Home Run calls. Two Point calls. Red Zone. Coming Out. Four minute offense. Two minute offense. Last Chance calls. Every situation that could happen...is covered.

And then when the time comes to make "the call"...there is no panic. There is no indecision. There is no hesitation, although it can sometimes be chaos on the field and in the stands. Although it can get rowdy and the air can get thick...there is a "refuge." That refuge is a peace...a peace that you have prepared. A peace that can feel like "arms" wrapped around you in support.

It is why coaches "do what they do." For times like these...when the game is on the line. Times that are late in the fourth. Times that call for one final drive. Time to get it done!

I had lunch today with one of my favorite coaches. We talked banking...beliefs...balance...and ball. He had been in the bank. We share a common belief. We talked about balance, both in competition and in life. We talked ball, pressure situations, and being prepared... in ball and in life. You know, fourth quarter stuff. Final drives.

Crystal's skin is looking like fourth quarter stuff. Her left side is burned, deeper in certain target areas. Fourth quarter burns. She continues to feel the effects of the radiation in other ways. Fatigue. Fourth quarter fatigue. Her hair is moving slowly, taking it's time coming back...but it is coming back. Just fourth quarter slow. Her side continues to hurt, regardless of the time of day or the position she is in. Fourth quarter pain.

Crystal has three more drives to make to the hospital...three final plays. Crystal has three final opportunities for the radiation to drive out the results of cancer in her body...three final plays. Crystal has a fourth quarter body...but with three more plays. Crystal is very late in the fourth...with a game plan in place...to destroy the enemy. Fourth quarter stuff...and one final drive.

In **Deuteronomy 33:27** is the following: *"The eternal God is your refuge, and underneath are the everlasting arms. He will drive out your enemy before you, saying "Destroy him!"*

Stand up and watch as Team Crystal makes a final drive. Watch as the enemy is destroyed! Watch...and enjoy...a drive to remember!

Driving home a point tonight...with "my view from the front."

– **Bill**

Fifty-One

Out of Bounds

Wednesday, March 10

Ever been there? You know, out of bounds? Ever seen...or heard someone else...who was clearly out of bounds. When you play for money, you need two feet inside the lines. When you are playing for the alumni, you only need one foot down. Too bad we can't make those same rules in life. Regardless of the rulebook you are using... there are still boundaries.

I would be the first to say that sometimes, in order to shake things up, you need to step across the lines. Be yourself. Let your hair down... oops, shouldn't have typed that. Or as Crystal said today, "You only live once." YOLO! However, sometimes stepping out of bounds can bring consequences.

Today on the phone, I had a customer who was "out of bounds." She wanted to imply...no, she was trying to tell me...how we do business. Whoa big fellow! I found it hard for her to know that when she is not an employee. I was patient. I was probably too kind. I bit my lip...for the good of the bank. What I wanted to say was

"Lady, you are out of bounds!" But don't worry, I took one for the team.

Let me give you a better example. Last week, Crystal came home from radiation with a story to tell. In this small waiting room before treatment, it was Crystal and two other women. One of the ladies was very prim and proper. She had been very reserved in her conversation. The other woman was, well, on the other end of the spectrum. Her conversation left nothing to be implied.

As the second woman began to get more detailed about her cancer and her treatments, she decided to do a "show and tell." Without hesitation she proceeded to show Crystal and "Lady Reserved" the results of radiation on her "girls"...her very large "girls"! And not just her "girls"...but the area underneath that was being treated as well. So, some heavy lifting had to take place in order for that area to be seen. (You got this picture yet?) Lady number two pulling out the "girls" for the girls to see. In broad daylight...and bigger than Dallas!

Now, "Lady Reserved" was rather quiet during the production. However, Crystal continued to nod and reply to the comments made by the lady who "had the floor." I am sure she was in shock! After the lesson had finished and the teacher had left the room, "Lady Reserved" told Crystal, "You should have seen your face when she pulled those out. Your eyes were as wide as saucers!" Now, somebody could easily have said in that room, "You're Out of Bounds!"

On the left side of Crystal's chest is drawn a boundary. Inside the lines, it continues to get more red with each trip to St. Vincent's. Some blisters have developed. The expensive lotion is not effective now as it needs to be. That radiation machine is powerful. The lines are there for a reason. Whatever you do...don't get "Out of Bounds!" (Unfortunately, now she knows what it is like to lay out topless!)

After today, we are down to two plays. Just like an offense using the boundary to stop the clock...Crystal has stepped out with just a little time on the clock. I think we have two plays left. Why not go for the end zone twice? Let it rip! We know the outcome...before the ball is snapped.

In the scriptures, Job took a while but finally figured out the outcome that awaited him. He realized the depth and magnitude of God's hand. In *Job 26:10* we find, *"He marks out the horizon on the face of the waters for a boundary between light and darkness."* What a comfort in knowing that our God not only placed physical boundaries on this earth but that we also have spiritual boundaries of protection when we are in His will. His lines are there for our good.

There is a lot of commotion on the sidelines. I am not sure if this entry had one foot down...or two feet...or no feet. Some will probably say I might have stepped "out of bounds." We may need to watch the replay of another angle to see. However, I do know this... without looking at the monitor. The clock has stopped for two more snaps.

The only angle I have...is "my view from the front!"
– Bill

Fifty-Two

Victory Formation

Thursday, March 11

As Crystal was making her next to last trip today for radiation, I was at a banking social, a.k.a. fish fry, with some potential customers. She was getting her flesh burned a little bit more...while I was pressing the flesh. She was one step closer to completing the task... while I was one step closer to completing the deal. She has one more opportunity to say "Good Bye" to the machine...while I am just getting started saying 'Welcome' to our bank. So ironic...

It is hard to shake a reputation. It is hard to not see people a certain way. When someone spends over twenty years doing something...that is usually what they are when in a crowd. So, today I was introduced as "Coach" by our Chairman of the Board. I consider that a great compliment considering whom it is coming from...and his background. I am just thankful there aren't many of us coaches in the bank. We really would have a financial crisis then.

I started the day this morning with a text coming in at 7:26 am from a coach friend of mine. Coaches like to put everything in a "game perspective." The text said, "Crystal has given herself a chance to win in the fourth. Now just win baby!" The first part came from my friend…from a long time ago. The last part was made famous by Al Davis, another famous football guy. Inspiration in a text. Words that I can relate to. Words that I can relay to Crystal. Words that I think of when I see her late at night or early in the morning.

My workday ended with another text coming in at 5:15 pm from another coach friend of mine. He too was looking through "coaching glasses." The text said, "Carry the ball with both hands and stay in bounds! They are out of time outs. Run clock run!" Something every coach knows is that when you are winning late…and they can't stop the clock…possession wins! Again, words a coach would understand. Words Crystal understands….as a coach's wife for so many years… and a cancer fighter for so many months.

As Team Crystal lines up for the last play tomorrow of a very hard fought game, I have two thoughts that will not leave my mind. Thoughts that I can relate to. Thoughts that maybe you can relate to as well. Two thoughts that are common to me at the end of a hard fought victory….and common to our family standing in support the entire game.

First is the "Victory Formation." That is the formation a football team uses when the game is won and they don't need to score any more points. The opponent has been defeated and there is enough time on the clock for one more play. (Listen to the crowd…)

The players come in tight. The quarterback is under center, flanked by two backs. There is one lone offensive player lined up about fifteen yards deep, as a security blanket, to just make sure. The quarterback takes the snap…and takes a knee! That is the best play in football, the best formation known to man. The game is won and it is time to enjoy...the Victory! (Listen to the crowd...)

The second thought is a verse of scripture found in *Psalm 95:6*, *"Come let us bow down in worship, let us kneel before The Lord our maker."* Another formation for us at the end of a hard fought victory! The enemy has been defeated. The Team is in tight...comfortable in the security that He has shown grace and mercy. (Listen to the praise...)

Tomorrow, Crystal and our family will take both of those positions. We will be in a Victory Formation...on our knees. From here on out, for the rest of her life, she will be associated as a cancer survivor! Introduced...as a cancer survivor! She can send the early morning text...to a teammate. (Listen... Listen... Listen to the Praise!)

"My view from the front"...with the clock showing 0:00.

– **Bill**

Fifty-Three

Remembering Mildred, Jarvis and Thomas

Thursday, March 25

Tomorrow will make two weeks since Crystal made her last trip to radiation treatment at St. Vincent's Hospital and The Bruno Cancer Center. Looking back, a lot can happen in two weeks. Skin can change...dogs can appear...and your mind can be refreshed. I will touch on a couple of those but first let me share with you the highlights of the last trip to treatment.

I took the day off on that Friday, March 12 in order to be with Crystal for her memorable last dose. As we were getting ready that morning for her assigned time, the phone rang...with bad news! The lady on the other end of the line said, "Mr. Gray, I'm sorry but the radiation machine is down today!" SAY WHAT?!!

She has not missed a single day for weeks...and TODAY the machine decides to not work! Remember the earlier reference to a game being "rained out?" This was ten times worse. "You don't understand, next week is Spring Break. We had this timed out just perfect. Today is the last day. FIX IT!"

Crystal had a scheduled appointment with her oncologist before she was to be radiated, so we went to that meeting...and prayed for "divine intervention." As we were leaving the consultation, a nurse from the radiation unit saw us in the hall. She was looking for another patient. The machine had been fixed!! She told Crystal if she was ready, she could jump in and get her last suntan. "Ready? Are you kidding me? Let's do it!"

Right place at the right time. We will never forget that day. Since that last treatment, Crystal's skin has continued to turn darker and darker. It is like when you get burned on the beach and then the next day pay for it...but much worse. More of a crimson or burgundy color. She also has several large blisters, or former blisters, from the concentration spots. They have exposed sensitive skin in those areas. This has also been a constant source of pain. She has gone through several tubes of those expensive creams. Yet, even with all this, she is glad her time under that machine is finished. She will never forget that feeling.

I have discovered that when you are married to a cancer survivor ...and have experienced what she has gone through...it is much harder to say "no." Therefore, in the last couple of weeks, we have taken some time off and relaxed in Orlando with just two children... and welcomed a new puppy into our house upon our return. The relaxation seems so far away now! I won't get started on my philosophy of dogs belonging outside. I do however remember what it was like for the last year or so...not to have to worry about a dog. I will never forget those quiet nights.

Finally, let me share one more memory. On that last day of radiation, we took some sweets from Edgar's Bakery to some special people. These people had the same expression of joy and hospitality on their faces every single time Crystal pulled up to the Cancer Center for radiation. "Good morning Crystal." "Hello Crystal." "How are you today Crystal?" "I'm praying for you Crystal." "Have a great day Crystal!" I mean, it was consistent. Regardless of how Crystal was feeling...it didn't matter to them. They were there for one reason and one reason only...to faithfully serve the patient...and park their car.

Mildred, Jarvis and Thomas were the valets that we got to know over the last several weeks. Something sweet doesn't come close to repaying them for the support they showed Crystal (and every other patient) each time she got out of the car. I don't think they were doing that service for sweets...but for The Lord. This may be the only place in Birmingham where your valet tells you he or she is praying for you...or for the man who just left ahead of you...and you believe every word he or she says.

Ephesians 6:7 describes their work ethic, *"Serve wholeheartedly, as if you were serving The Lord, not men."* We would all be better off if we took that approach on a more consistent basis in our daily lives. There have been so many people, places, and things that we will remember when we look back at this experience one day. None will be more clear than those three individuals in their khaki shirts, sometimes in the rain...the heat...and even the snow...parking cars and praying away cancer. Faces we both will never forget.

Rubbing on cream...and picking up puppy poop...while keeping "my view from the front."

– Bill

Fifty-Four

July 2014

Celebrating 5!

On July 16, 2014, Crystal celebrated "beating cancer for 5 years!" As part of her "surprise party," I have put this book together. The past 53 Chapters you have just read is an accumulation of the journey she and our family took over a period of eight months from July 2009 to March 2010. A period of time in the Gray family that we will never forget.

Crystal has now graduated from having a check-up with the oncologist every three months to every six months. Her numbers continue to look good. As any Cancer survivor will tell you...5 years is a landmark moment. However, as her doctor told me early on in this journey, "Crystal will always be a survivor regardless of the time down the road."

But Doc, what if it comes back?

Her reply, "Bill, if the horse gets out of the barn a second time... there isn't much we can do."

I've never owned a horse. I have been on one or two. I've never built a barn. I do like to see them out the side window riding through the country side of Tennessee...or Alabama...or Mississippi. Horses. Barns. Nothing we can do.

What she was saying, in her own way, was that the future is not in our hands. Deep spiritual truths...while drawing a comparison with the lodging arrangements of an equine. Quoting scripture...without opening the Word.

The children have all added five years to their age since this journey began. In many ways, they continue to be the best motivation in Crystal's daily battle with cancer. Motivation to take the "prescription drug that is as close as you can get to chemo." One that she still takes daily...and will for many years to come.

Motivation to cope with the fact that she has eliminated every ounce and inch of anything in her body that would be associated with estrogen. Estrogen isn't good...when you have a cancer that thrives on estrogen. Motivation to face the reality that she can't take the normal hormone pills because it would increase the chances of her cancer coming back. Because of the children...and now grandchildren...Crystal continues to press on. What else would you expect?

Let's consider *James 4:13-15, "Now listen, you who say, 'Today or tomorrow we will go to this or that city, spend a year there, carry on business and make money.' Why, you do not even know what will happen tomorrow. What is your life? You are a mist that appears for a little while and then vanishes. Instead, you ought to say, 'If it is the Lord's will, we will live and do this or that.'"*

No horses. No barns. Just a reminder that we just don't know. We don't really know about today...or tomorrow. What we do know is that in the grand scheme, life is short. If The Lord allows any of us to live through today...or into tomorrow...we all need to "do this or that!"

The "this" and the "that" is making sure each of us have a relationship with Jesus Christ...a personal relationship. It is making sure those around us that we love dearly...know Him as well. It is what we all should be busy about...regardless of our health, either good or bad.

Each time that happens...there is another Reason To Celebrate!!

This is the most important reminder...from this journey...from this season in our life...from "my view from the front."

– Bill

Many Thanks to the following...

To Brittany, Briana, Austin, Payton and Bailey...Thank you team for all the love you have shown your mother during this battle with cancer. Know that each of you are the inspiration for your mother to press on. I can't tell you how many times she has cried thinking of the things she may miss in your lives. Each in your own way has been there for her...at just the right time. Our quiver is certainly full...of love.

To Justin and Wesley...You guys have joined our family and pledged to take care of two of our daughters. You have both provided comfort for our girls during this time in their life. You have also given Crystal and I the comfort in knowing that Brittany and Briana have married men who are putting Jesus first in your homes. Who could want more?

To Gray and John Warren...You two have made CeCe and Bops proud grandparents. Joy comes to our heart every time we see your face or hear your voice. Thanks for giving your mom's mom more reason to fight this disease.

To our extended families, the Crosby's and the Gray's...Thank you for all the many ways you have loved us through the years. We hold dear the times each of you have prayed for Crystal and our family. Support from the family has always been a given...a hedge of protection!

To our Bible Study class, the "Muddler's," at Green Valley Baptist Church...Thanks to each of you for rising up and going above and beyond what we could ever have imagined. In your own special way you have lifted Crystal up...picked up the slack with the children... and made sure we had food, food, and more food. You are a special group and we will always be reminded of the way that you loved on the Gray's.

To our church family at GVBC...Words can't describe the warmth Crystal has felt from your caring hearts. We have seen it in your eyes...and your actions. Thank you for being our extended family during so many long weeks.

To our friends and prayer warriors, literally all over the country... Crystal has said on many occasions through this journey that she "feels the strength and comfort of those praying for her." Many of you we have known for a long time, while others we only know you by a name on CaringBridge. However, each one of you will always be special in our hearts. From driving for hours just to be a face we could see...to showing us in living color the places Crystal's name has been lifted up...to walking into a waiting room with an armful of Milo's hamburgers...to making sure a day didn't go by without a word of encouragement...to cheesy noodle soup...to making sure we "had what we need"...to loving on our kids and getting their minds on something else for a time. We will never be able to adequately say "thank you." You will never know what you have meant to each one of the Gray's.

And finally, to our pastor...Thank you for reminding us every

Sunday, that we have a BIG GOD. A God who loves us. A God who cares for us. A God who is in control. Thank you for showing us that it really isn't about us...but about those around us lost without a relationship with Jesus Christ. There is indeed no "plan B." That is why it is important for all of us to remember...with or without cancer...this is the only shot at life we get.

Let's Celebrate His Love!